BLADDER CANCER

A Patient-Friendly Guide to Understanding Your Diagnosis and Treatment Options

David Pulver

Bladder Cancer Survivor

Mark Schoenberg, MD

University Professor & Chairman
Department of Urology
Montefiore Medical Center and
Albert Einstein College of Medicine
Bronx, New York

Fran Pulver

Health Writer and Cancer Survivor

with Risa Alberts

PFP

Patient-Friendly Publishing

Cover and interior design by Suzanne Albertson, *suzannealbertson.com*
Medical illustrations by Caitlin Duckwall, Dragonfly Media Group
Digital book(s) (epub and mobi) produced by *Booknook.biz*

This book is not intended to be a substitute for professional medical advice and should not be used to diagnose or treat any medical condition. For diagnosis or treatment of any medical condition, consult your own physician. For the diagnosis or treatment of any medical condition, always seek the advice of your physician or other qualified health care professional. The information in this book is intended solely for informational purposes and should not be construed as medical advice. As such, the reader assumes full responsibility for the appropriate use of the medical and health information contained in this book and agrees to hold the authors and publisher and any of its third-party providers harmless from any and all claims or action arising from the use or reliance on any of the information contained in this book. The authors and publisher disclaim liability for any medical outcomes that may occur as a result of the use or reliance on the medical or health information contained in this book.

The authors and publisher have made every effort to provide accurate information. However, they are not responsible for errors, omissions, or any outcomes related to the use of the contents of this book and take no responsibility for the use of the products and procedures described. Always seek the advice of your physician or other qualified health care provider with any questions you may have regarding a medical condition or treatment and before embarking on any medical program or treatment. Never disregard professional medical advice or delay seeking professional medical advice because of something you have read in this book.

All resources provided in this book are for informational purposes only and do not constitute endorsement of any websites, web pages, or other sources. Readers should be aware that the websites and web pages referred to or listed in this book are subject to change. The authors and publisher have no control over and take no responsibility for third-party websites or web pages or their content.

Library of Congress cataloging information forthcoming.

ISBN: 978-1-946364-00-5 (paperback)
ISBN: 978-1-946364-01-2 (hardcover)
ISBN: 978-1-946364-02-9 (Kindle)
ISBN: 978-1-946364-03-6 (EPUB)

Patient-Friendly Publishing
Website: *www.bladdercancerbook.org*
E-mail: *bladdercancerbook@gmail.com*

Printed in the United States of America

*This book is dedicated to the more than 79,000 people in
this country who are diagnosed with bladder cancer each year,
to the more than 696,000 people in this country currently living with
this disease, and to the countless family members, friends,
and others who love and care for them.*

CONTENTS

Illustrations   x

Preface: A Doctor-Patient Partnership   xi
  From a Patient's Perspective by David Pulver,   xi
    bladder cancer survivor
  From a Doctor's Perspective by Mark Schoenberg, MD   xiii
About the Authors   xv
Acknowledgments   xvii

PART 1   WHAT ALL PATIENTS NEED TO KNOW

CHAPTER 1:
Introduction   3
What You Will Learn from This Book   4

CHAPTER 2:
How to Become a Proactive Patient   9
Understanding the "Language" of Bladder Cancer   9
Understanding Your Diagnosis   10
Choosing Your Doctors   11
Choosing Your Treatment Facilities   14
Understanding Your Treatment Options   15
Preparing for Your Doctor's Appointments   16
Using the Internet   17
Keeping Records of Your Bladder Cancer History   18

CHAPTER 3:
An Introduction to the Urinary System   21
The Urinary System   21
The Prostate, Urinary Sphincters, and Lymph Nodes   30

CHAPTER 4:

Diagnosing Bladder Cancer: Procedures and Tests   33

Cystoscopy	36
Urine Tests	38
Imaging Tests	39
TURBT	44
Blue Light Cystoscopy	46
Use of Diagnostic Procedures and Tests After Initial Diagnosis	47

CHAPTER 5:

Understanding Your Bladder Cancer Diagnosis   49

What Is the Grade of My Bladder Cancer?	49
What Is the Stage of My Bladder Cancer?	50
What Is the Cell Type of My Bladder Cancer?	52
What Does My Bladder Cancer Diagnosis Mean?	53
What Are My Risks of Recurrence and/or Progression?	55
Should I Get a Second Opinion?	57

PART 2	TREATMENTS FOR NON-MUSCLE-INVASIVE BLADDER CANCER

CHAPTER 6:

Non-Muscle-Invasive Bladder Cancer   61

What Are the Stages of Non-Muscle-Invasive Bladder Cancer?	62
What Are the Grades of Non-Muscle-Invasive Bladder Cancer?	62
What Are the Risks of Recurrence and/or Progression of Non-Muscle-Invasive Bladder Cancer?	63
How Is Non-Muscle-Invasive Bladder Cancer Treated?	63
Ta, CIS, and T1 Tumors: What You Need to Know	68
How Is Non-Muscle-Invasive Bladder Cancer Monitored?	71

PART 3   TREATMENTS FOR MUSCLE-INVASIVE BLADDER CANCER

CHAPTER 7:

Introduction to Muscle-Invasive Bladder Cancer   75

What Are the Stages of Muscle-Invasive Bladder Cancer?   75
What Is the Grade of Muscle-Invasive Bladder Cancer?   76
What Are the Treatment Options for Muscle-Invasive   77
   Bladder Cancer?

CHAPTER 8:

The Decision to Have a Radical Cystectomy   79

When Is a Radical Cystectomy Indicated?   80
Who Is a Candidate for a Radical Cystectomy?   80
What Is Involved in the Decision to Have a Radical Cystectomy?   81
What Are the Benefits of a Radical Cystectomy?   82
What Are the Risks of a Radical Cystectomy?   83
What Are the Other Treatment Options?   83

CHAPTER 9:

Undergoing a Radical Cystectomy   85

Preparing for a Radical Cystectomy   85
What Is Involved in Undergoing a Radical Cystectomy?   89
Your Postoperative Pathology Report   93

CHAPTER 10:

Choosing a Urinary Tract Reconstruction   95

Ileal Conduit   96
Orthotopic Neobladder   99
Continent Catheterizable Reservoir   103
Choosing a Surgeon   106
Talking with Other Patients   106

CHAPTER 11:

Recovery After a Radical Cystectomy   **109**

Your Postoperative Hospital Stay   109
When You Get Home — the Road to Recovery   113
Follow-up Care After a Radical Cystectomy   115
Impact of a Radical Cystectomy on Sexual Function and Fertility   116
For Patients with An Ileal Conduit: Caring for Your Stoma   119

CHAPTER 12:

Bladder Preservation Therapy   **123**

Who Is a Good Candidate for Bladder Preservation Therapy?   123
The Decision to Have Bladder Preservation Therapy   127
Bladder Preservation Therapy: A Three-Pronged Approach   129
What Is the Follow-up Care After Bladder Preservation Therapy?   131
What Are the Side Effects of Bladder Preservation Therapy?   132

PART 4   TREATMENTS FOR METASTATIC BLADDER CANCER

CHAPTER 13:

Metastatic Bladder Cancer   **135**

How Is Metastatic Bladder Cancer Diagnosed?   135
What Is the Staging System for Metastatic Bladder Cancer?   136
What You Need to Know About Systemic Chemotherapy   137
Immunotherapy as a Treatment for Metastatic Bladder Cancer   144
Are Clinical Trials an Option for Metastatic Bladder Cancer?   144
When Is Radiation Therapy Used?   146
What Is Palliative Care?   146

PART 5   SURVIVORSHIP

CHAPTER 14:

Bladder Cancer Survivorship   **149**

When Active Treatment Ends — New Questions and Concerns   149
Creating a Survivorship Care Plan   152
Tips for Taking a Proactive Role in Your Follow-up Care   155

PART 6   APPENDIXES

A. Bladder Cancer Risk Factors   161

B. Bladder Cancer Health Care Professionals   163

C. Bladder Cancer Resources   167

D. Glossary of Bladder Cancer Terms   175

Index   193

ILLUSTRATIONS

FIGURES

3.1 Male Urinary Tract (front view)	22
3.2 Male Lower Urinary Tract (side view)	22
3.3 Female Urinary Tract (front view)	23
3.4 Female Lower Urinary Tract (side view)	23
3.5 Kidneys	24
3.6 Male Bladder	26
3.7 Female Bladder	27
3.8 Layers of the Bladder Wall	28
3.9 Lymph Nodes	31
4.1 Cystoscopy	36
4.2 TURBT	44
5.1 Stages of Bladder Cancer	50
5.2 The TNM Staging System for Bladder Cancer	51
6.1 Stages of Non-Muscle-Invasive Bladder Cancer	62
6.2 Intravesical Drug Therapy	66
7.1 Stages of Muscle-Invasive Bladder Cancer	76
8.1 Survival Rates by Stage After a Radical Cystectomy	82
10.1 Ileal Conduit	97
10.2 Orthotopic Neobladder	100
10.3 Continent Catheterizable Reservoir	104

PREFACE: A DOCTOR-PATIENT PARTNERSHIP

From a Patient's Perspective
by David Pulver, bladder cancer survivor

When you first learn you have bladder cancer, you feel frightened, vulnerable, and very much in need of help. Most people go to their computer and Google the words "bladder cancer," and up pops more information than they can imagine. They start clicking away, and they get even more frightened, confused, and depressed. They wonder how they are going to make sense of all the information. They try to understand how this avalanche of information applies to their own situation.

I fully understand these feelings. I experienced them myself in August 2007 when I first learned I had bladder cancer. When I expressed my frustration to Dr. Mark Schoenberg, my doctor at Johns Hopkins, he gave me a copy of his book, *The Guide to Living with Bladder Cancer*. It was published in 2000 but was out of print. I read the book and found that it provided the best bladder cancer information available at the time.

When I learned that Dr. Schoenberg was working with some of the best bladder cancer doctors in the United States and Canada to revise and update his book, I wanted to help. I offered to help fund the project and to provide input with respect to making the writing style more patient-friendly. Eventually, I became personally involved in the writing of the book. My sister, Fran Pulver, a professional health and medical writer and thirteen-year cancer survivor, joined in this effort.

The publication of *Bladder Cancer: A Patient-Friendly Guide to Understanding Your Diagnosis and Treatment Options* is the culmination of this collaborative effort. The book combines expert medical information with a clear writing style that presents and organizes the information in the most patient-friendly way. The mission of the book is to educate patients about bladder cancer so they can understand their diagnosis and make informed decisions regarding their treatment and care.

As a ten-year bladder cancer survivor, I have become very involved in the bladder cancer community. I joined the Board of Directors of BCAN (Bladder Cancer Advocacy Network, *bcan.org*), a wonderful nonprofit advocacy organization for bladder cancer patients. Founded in 2005 by Diane Zipursky Quale and the late John Quale, BCAN is dedicated to educating patients and their families about bladder cancer, funding bladder cancer research, advocating for bladder cancer research, and raising public awareness about the disease. I also counsel many bladder cancer patients and help them think through their bladder cancer situation. These experiences, in addition to my own experience as a survivor of a serious form of bladder cancer, have helped me understand how the patient thinks and what they want to know.

This book project has been a labor of love. It is my hope and dream that patients diagnosed with bladder cancer will benefit from this book.

Any profits realized from this book will be donated to bladder cancer research.

From a Doctor's Perspective
by Mark Schoenberg, MD

David Pulver became a patient of mine in 2007. From the beginning, I could tell David was a different kind of patient. He had an insatiable thirst for knowledge about bladder cancer. He wanted to better understand his disease and participate in his treatment decisions. He had searched the Internet and was not satisfied with the information available about bladder cancer.

I gave David a copy of *The Guide to Living with Bladder Cancer,* a book published in 2000, which I wrote with my colleagues at Johns Hopkins and was out of print at the time. David found the book to be the most useful information about bladder cancer he had read to that point. Yet, there were aspects of the book he thought could be improved. I told David that I was working with some of the best bladder cancer doctors in the U.S. and Canada to update the book. David was very excited about the project and made a significant financial contribution to help fund the book.

As David kept abreast of the progress of the book, he became increasingly concerned that the manuscript was not meeting his vision for the book. His idea was to marry the best medical information on bladder cancer with a clear, concise, patient-friendly writing style. David's concept of patient-friendly writing was greatly influenced by his experience as a bladder cancer survivor, his work as a member of the Board of Directors of BCAN (Bladder Cancer Advocacy Network, *bcan.org*), and his experience counseling many patients diagnosed with bladder cancer.

Ultimately, David became one of the authors of the book. He enlisted the help of his sister, Fran Pulver, a professional health and medical writer and thirteen-year cancer survivor. The combination of the medical input from many fine bladder cancer doctors, together with relentless efforts by David and Fran to present the information in the most patient-friendly way, has resulted in a terrific book that I believe every person who is diagnosed with bladder cancer will find extremely useful.

ABOUT THE AUTHORS

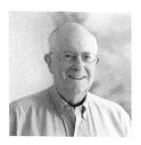

David Pulver is a ten-year survivor of a serious form of bladder cancer. He has served on the Board of Directors of BCAN (Bladder Cancer Advocacy Network, *bcan.org*) since 2008. BCAN is dedicated to increasing public awareness of bladder cancer, advancing research directed toward bladder cancer, and educating and supporting bladder cancer patients and their families. David is President of Cornerstone Capital, Inc., a private investment company. Prior to starting Cornerstone Capital, he co-founded and was Chairman and Co-CEO of The Children's Place, a leading retailer of children's clothing. David serves on the Board of Directors of Carter's, a leading manufacturer and retailer of infants and young children's apparel. He previously served on the Board of Directors of Costco Wholesale and on the Board of Directors of the Public Health Research Institute, a leading nonprofit medical research organization specializing in infectious diseases. David serves on the Board of Trustees of Colby College, located in Waterville, Maine. He earned his BA from Colby College and his MBA from Harvard Business School. David lives in Palm Beach Gardens, Florida, with his wife Carol.

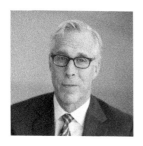

Mark Schoenberg, **MD**, is University Professor & Chairman of the Department of Urology at the Montefiore Medical Center and the Albert Einstein College of Medicine, Bronx, New York. Dr. Schoenberg obtained his MD degree from the University of Texas (Houston) and his training in Surgery and Urology at the University of Pennsylvania (Philadelphia). Under the auspices of the American Cancer Society, Dr. Schoenberg served as a fellow in urologic oncology at The James Buchanan Brady Urological Institute of The Johns Hopkins University (Baltimore). He subsequently joined the Hopkins faculty and rose to the rank of Professor and Director of Urologic Oncology. Dr. Schoenberg is an internationally acknowledged authority on the management of urothelial cancer and is the author or coauthor of over 170 articles in the peer-reviewed literature. He has served on the editorial staffs of the peer-reviewed journals

Urologic Oncology, The Journal of Urology, and *Urology.* He is the author of *The Guide to Living with Bladder Cancer (2000).* He is an editor of the *Textbook of Bladder Cancer* (2006), a past contributor to *Campbell's Urology* (2008), and an editor of *Bladder Cancer: Diagnosis and Clinical Management* (2015).

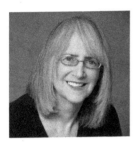 **Fran Pulver** has worked as a health and medical writer since 1991. She has written articles for Harvard Medical School's *Harvard Heart Letter* and *Better Health for Life* and contributed to *A Guide to Alzheimer's Disease,* published by Harvard Health Publications. She is the author of the *Guide to Getting the Best Cancer Treatment* and the *Guide to Getting the Best Healthcare,* published by PinnacleCare. Fran has over 25 years of experience writing health and medical content for health care providers, health publications, and websites. She writes consumer-friendly content that helps patients become actively involved in decisions about their health care. In addition to medical writing, she has copyedited or proofread more than 300 academic books and journals for university presses and scientific publishers. Fran is a thirteen-year cancer survivor and drew from her personal experience in coauthoring this book. A resident of Cambridge, Massachusetts, she currently works as a freelance writer, editor, and proofreader.

ACKNOWLEDGMENTS

David Pulver, Dr. Mark Schoenberg, and Fran Pulver want to acknowledge and thank the following people for their contributions to this book.

Patients

The many patients David counseled — who helped him better understand the problems, questions, and needs of people diagnosed with bladder cancer.

Doctors

Trinity Bivalacqua, MD, Johns Hopkins University, Baltimore, MD
Bernard Bochner, MD, Memorial Sloan Kettering Cancer Center, New York, NY
Sam Chang, MD, Vanderbilt University, Nashville, TN
Michael Cookson, MD, University of Oklahoma, Oklahoma City, OK
Sia Daneshmand, MD, USC Institute of Urology, Los Angeles, CA
Theodore DeWeese, MD, Johns Hopkins University, Baltimore, MD
Colin Dinney, MD, MD Anderson Cancer Center, Houston, TX
Mario Eisenberger, MD, Johns Hopkins University, Baltimore, MD
Jonathan Epstein, MD, Johns Hopkins University, Baltimore, MD
Elliot Fishman, MD, Johns Hopkins University, Baltimore, MD
Barton Grossman, MD, MD Anderson Cancer Center, Houston, TX
Thomas Guzzo, MD, Hospital of the University of Pennsylvania, Philadelphia, PA
Niall Heney, MD, Massachusetts General Hospital, Boston, MA
Ashish Kamat, MD, MD Anderson Cancer Center, Houston, TX
Adam Kibel, MD, Brigham and Women's Hospital, Boston, MA
Donald Lamm, MD, BCG Oncology, Phoenix, AZ
Cheryl Lee, MD, Ohio State University, Columbus, OH
Seth Lerner, MD, Baylor College of Medicine, Houston, TX
Jen-Jane Liu, MD, Oregon Health & Science University, Portland, OR
Edward Messing, MD, University of Rochester, Rochester, NY
Matthew Milowsky, MD, University of North Carolina, Chapel Hill, NC
George Netto, MD, UAB School of Medicine, Birmingham, AL

Matthew Nielsen, MD, University of North Carolina, Chapel Hill, NC
Dorothy Rosenthal, MD, Johns Hopkins University, Baltimore, MD
William Shipley, MD, Massachusetts General Hospital, Boston, MA
Angela Smith, MD, University of North Carolina, Chapel Hill, NC
Norm Smith, MD, University of Chicago, Chicago, IL
Gary Steinberg, MD, University of Chicago, Chicago, IL
Cora Sternberg, MD, San Camillo-Forlanini Hospital, Rome, Italy

Enterostomal Therapy (ET) Nurse

Joanne Walker, RN, Johns Hopkins University, Baltimore, MD, who made a significant contribution to the book on the topic of ostomy care.

Content Development

Risa Alberts, who provided invaluable assistance with content development.

Patient Advocate

Diane Zipursky Quale, co-founder of BCAN (Bladder Cancer Advocacy Network), the leading bladder cancer patient advocacy organization in the United States.

Medical Illustrator

Caitlin Duckwall, Dragonfly Media Group, who did a splendid job of producing the medical illustrations.

Book Designer

Suzanne Albertson, who went beyond the call of duty to design a terrific book cover and interior design.

E-Book Conversion

Kimberly ("Hitch") Hitchens, owner of Booknook.biz, whose expertise and support was invaluable in converting the print book to a terrific e-book.

Publishing Consultant

Shirley Spence, who guided us through the publishing process.

Part 1 consists of **Chapters 1–5,** which provide general information all bladder cancer patients need to know to understand their diagnosis and take an active role in their care. After reading these chapters, you may then choose to read only the remaining chapter or chapters that are applicable to your specific diagnosis.

Chapter 1 describes what you will learn from this book, which is intended to help you and your family become active, informed participants in decisions about your treatment and care. **Chapter 2** discusses skills and strategies you can learn to become your own advocate in fighting your disease. **Chapter 3** discusses the anatomy and functions of the bladder and other organs of the urinary system. **Chapter 4** focuses on the diagnostic tools used to diagnose bladder cancer. **Chapter 5** presents key information you need to know to understand your diagnosis.

CHAPTER 1

Introduction

When you first learn you have bladder cancer, you most likely feel frightened, uninformed, and unprepared to deal with the disease. You hear only the word *cancer* and nothing else. Your first thought may be that the disease is fatal and your days are numbered. Many scenarios and questions start running through your mind: How long will I live? Was the cancer caught in time? Can I be cured? What treatments will I need, and how will they affect my work and family life? What can I do to make sure I get the best possible cancer care and treatment outcomes?

To grapple with these questions, you need to understand your diagnosis and treatment options, and how your cancer and its treatment will affect you and your family. You need your doctor to explain in clear language the facts about your medical condition and discuss your treatment options. You also need the support of family and friends to help gather and absorb this information and formulate questions. Only by gaining an understanding of your disease can you become an active partner with your health care providers and participate in making decisions about your cancer treatment and care.

THE MISSION OF THIS BOOK

The mission of this book is to educate patients about bladder cancer so they can understand their diagnosis and make informed decisions regarding their treatment and care.

Fortunately, the majority of patients diagnosed with bladder cancer have a highly treatable form of the disease that, with proper medical management, is usually not life threatening. However, about 25% of patients are diagnosed with more advanced stages of bladder cancer, requiring them to undergo complex therapies that are potentially life changing. Regardless of the challenges you and your loved ones encounter during your cancer journey, taking a proactive role in your care will increase the likelihood of getting the best possible outcomes for your disease.

BLADDER CANCER STATISTICS FOR THE UNITED STATES

Bladder cancer is the fifth most common cancer in the United States, with more than 696,000 men and women living with a history of the disease. About 90% of people diagnosed with bladder cancer are age 55 years and older, and the average age at the time of diagnosis is 73. The incidence of bladder cancer is about 4 times higher in men than in women. In men, bladder cancer is the fourth most common cancer and the ninth most common cause of cancer death. In women, bladder cancer is the twelfth most common cancer and the fifteenth most common cause of cancer death. The American Cancer Society estimated there would be about 79,030 new cases of bladder cancer (60,490 in men and 18,540 in women) and about 16,870 deaths from bladder cancer (12,240 in men and 4,630 in women) in the United States in 2017. Despite the prevalence of bladder cancer, there is a relative lack of public awareness about this disease compared to other common cancers such as breast cancer, colon cancer, and prostate cancer.

What You Will Learn from This Book

This book is a patients' guide to understanding and living with bladder cancer. It is written for the benefit of people who are diagnosed with this disease and for the friends and loved ones who want to support them on their cancer journey. The book is intended to be a useful guide from the moment you are diagnosed with bladder cancer. Because the book is designed to be patient-friendly, it is written in plain and simple language. All medical terminology and concepts are translated into vocabulary that can be easily understood by the general reader.

Becoming an educated, proactive patient will enable you to make informed decisions about your treatment and care and, as a result, optimize your chance of getting the best possible outcomes for your disease. With these goals in mind, this book provides information, tools, and resources that will help you select the right doctors, understand your diagnosis and treatment options, partner with your medical team, and be your own advocate throughout your cancer journey.

This book is organized into 6 parts, consisting of 14 chapters and 4 appendixes. We recommend you first read Part 1 (chapters 1–5), which provides information all patients with bladder cancer need to know. Part 1 includes information on becoming a proactive patient, the anatomy and functions of the urinary system, how bladder cancer is diagnosed, and what you need to know to understand your diagnosis.

The next step is to read the chapter or chapters that discuss the treatment options for your specific diagnosis. Part 2 (chapter 6) discusses the treatments for *non-muscle-invasive* bladder cancer. Part 3 (chapters 7–12) discusses the treatments for *muscle-invasive* bladder cancer. Part 4 (chapter 13) discusses the treatments for *metastatic* bladder cancer.

Part 5 (chapter 14) discusses challenges facing bladder cancer survivors — particularly when transitioning from active treatment to follow-up care. Finally, Part 6 consists of 4 appendixes, including a glossary and list of additional resources.

The following is an overview of the topics covered in this book:

PART 1 • WHAT ALL PATIENTS NEED TO KNOW

Chapter 1 — Introduction (this chapter).

Chapter 2 — How to Become a Proactive Patient discusses how to take an active role in your cancer care and be your own advocate. Taking control of your medical care is key to getting the best possible outcomes for your disease.

Chapter 3 — An Introduction to the Urinary System describes the anatomy and functions of the urinary system. It is a geography lesson on the parts of the body that you need to know about as you read this book.

Chapter 4 — Diagnosing Bladder Cancer: Procedures and Tests describes the diagnostic tools used to diagnose bladder cancer.

Chapter 5 — Understanding Your Bladder Cancer Diagnosis discusses the information you need to know to understand your diagnosis, including the stages and grades of bladder cancer. Getting a complete and accurate diagnosis is a prerequisite for determining your treatment options.

PART 2 • TREATMENTS FOR NON-MUSCLE-INVASIVE BLADDER CANCER

Chapter 6 — Non-Muscle-Invasive Bladder Cancer discusses the different stages and grades of non-muscle-invasive bladder cancer and its treatment.

PART 3 • TREATMENTS FOR MUSCLE-INVASIVE BLADDER CANCER

Chapter 7 — Muscle-Invasive Bladder Cancer discusses the stages and grade of muscle-invasive bladder cancer and includes an overview of its treatment. The different treatment options for muscle-invasive bladder cancer are discussed at length in chapters 8–12.

Chapter 8 — The Decision to Have a Radical Cystectomy discusses factors you need to consider when deciding if a radical cystectomy is right for you. A *radical cystectomy* is a surgical procedure that removes the bladder and reconstructs the lower urinary tract to create a way for urine to be eliminated from the body after the bladder is removed. A radical cystectomy is considered the "gold standard" treatment for muscle-invasive bladder cancer.

Chapter 9 — Undergoing a Radical Cystectomy discusses how to prepare for a radical cystectomy, what is involved in the surgical procedure, and what you will learn from your postoperative pathology report.

Chapter 10 — Choosing a Urinary Tract Reconstruction discusses the different types of urinary tract reconstructions for patients undergoing a radical cystectomy, and what you need to know to decide which type of urinary tract reconstruction is best for you.

Chapter 11 — Recovery After a Radical Cystectomy discusses recovery from a radical cystectomy during your postoperative hospital stay and after you leave the hospital to continue your recovery and resume your normal daily activities.

Chapter 12 — Bladder Preservation Therapy discusses a possible alternative to a radical cystectomy for selected patients. *Bladder preservation therapy* — also called *bladder-sparing therapy* or *trimodality therapy (TMT)* — treats bladder cancer without removing the bladder.

PART 4 · TREATMENTS FOR METASTATIC BLADDER CANCER

Chapter 13 — Metastatic Bladder Cancer discusses the treatment of bladder cancer that has spread outside the bladder to the lymph nodes and/or distant parts of the body. The primary treatment for metastatic bladder cancer is systemic chemotherapy.

PART 5 · SURVIVORSHIP

Chapter 14 — Bladder Cancer Survivorship discusses the transition from active treatment to follow-up care, including what should be included in a survivorship care plan.

PART 6 • APPENDIXES

Appendix A — Bladder Cancer Risk Factors discusses the factors that increase the risk of developing bladder cancer.

Appendix B — Bladder Cancer Health Care Professionals is a list of the different health care professionals and the roles they play in caring for patients with bladder cancer.

Appendix C — Bladder Cancer Resources is a list of organizations and websites that offer educational materials, support, and advocacy for people diagnosed with bladder cancer and their families and friends.

Appendix D — Glossary of Bladder Cancer Terms translates complex medical terms into easy-to-understand language.

NOTE TO THE READER

The information in this book is intended solely for informational purposes and should never be used as a substitute for the advice of a medical professional. Do not base your diagnosis and/or treatment options on anything you read in this book. This book was written to help you participate in an ongoing doctor-patient dialogue, so you can take an active role in your treatment and care.

The information in this book is not a substitute for professional medical care and should not be used for the diagnosis or treatment of any medical condition. Always talk to your doctor before embarking on a course of treatment or making any changes in your care. Never disregard professional medical advice or delay seeking professional medical advice because of something you read in this book.

CHAPTER 2

How to Become a Proactive Patient

To increase the likelihood that you get the best possible outcomes for your disease, it is important that you take a proactive role in your care.

This chapter discusses the following strategies for becoming a proactive patient:

- Understanding the "language" of bladder cancer
- Understanding your diagnosis
- Choosing your doctors
- Choosing your treatment facilities
- Understanding your treatment options
- Preparing for your doctor's appointments
- Using the Internet
- Keeping records of your bladder cancer history

Understanding the "Language" of Bladder Cancer

As you start learning about bladder cancer, you will quickly realize that you need to learn new words, such as *cystoscopy, TURBT (transurethral resection of bladder tumor), cytology, stage, grade, intravesical drug therapy, radical cystectomy, progression*, and *urothelium*. Becoming familiar with relevant medical terms is an important step in demystifying your disease and educating yourself so you can play an active role in decisions impacting your treatment and care.

To acquaint you with the specialized language used by doctors to discuss bladder cancer — and which may appear in your medical reports and test results — medical terms are translated into easy-to-understand language throughout the book. There is also a glossary of terms related to bladder cancer in appendix D, "Glossary of Bladder Cancer Terms."

Understanding Your Diagnosis

Understanding your diagnosis is key to making informed treatment decisions (see chapter 5). You will need your doctor to explain, in plain language, your diagnosis and what it means. Absorbing this information usually takes time and effort, but it is time and energy well spent.

Questions you need to ask your doctor about your diagnosis include the following:

- What is the *grade* of my bladder cancer?
- What is the *stage* of my bladder cancer?
- What is the *cell type* of my bladder cancer?
- What is the *prognosis* for my bladder cancer?
- What are the risks of *recurrence* and/or *progression*?

YOUR RELATIONSHIP WITH YOUR DOCTOR IS KEY

Communication is key to building a good relationship with your doctor. You need a doctor who answers all your questions in clear language and engages in conversations about your issues and concerns. You need to be able to communicate with your doctor about your treatment goals, your tolerance for risk, your values, and your needs. It is important that your relationship with your doctor is based on mutual trust and respect, and that you feel like you are being treated in a caring and compassionate manner.

Choosing Your Doctors

During a routine physical examination, your primary care doctor may detect blood in your urine, called *hematuria* — which is the most common symptom of bladder cancer. Most doctors who evaluate hematuria or other symptoms of bladder cancer start by performing two laboratory tests — a urinalysis and a urine culture — to determine if there is a urinary tract infection, which is often the cause of the symptoms. Other causes of the symptoms include benign conditions, such as kidney stones, or blood-thinning medications. If based on these tests, you do not have a urinary tract infection and there is no other explanation for your symptoms, you should be evaluated for bladder cancer by a general urologist, a doctor who specializes in treating diseases of the urinary tract. If you do not have a general urologist, you can ask your primary care doctor for a referral.

A ***general urologist*** is a doctor who has completed residency training in general urology but does not specialize in bladder cancer. A general urologist has the surgical training and experience to perform initial diagnostic evaluations of patients with bladder cancer and to treat common forms of the disease. If you are diagnosed with a more advanced form of bladder cancer or want a second opinion, you should consult with a ***urologic oncologist***, a doctor who specializes in treating urologic cancers, including bladder cancer. In addition to residency training in general urology, urologic oncologists generally have completed multi-year fellowship programs involving advanced surgical training and medical education about urologic cancers. Urologic oncologists usually practice at major medical centers.

Both general urologists and urologic oncologists diagnose and treat bladder cancer. In choosing your doctors, which type of doctor to see is usually based on the form of bladder cancer you have and the treatment you need.

If you are looking for a urologic oncologist, the following are ways to find one:

- Ask your general urologist or primary care doctor for recommendations.
- Look for a urologic oncologist at an NCI-designated cancer center(s) of your choice. There are 69 NCI-designated cancer centers in 35 states and the District of Columbia. You can find links to the

websites of NCI-designated cancer centers closest to your area by going online to *http://cancercenters.cancer.gov/center/cancercenters*. Once on the NCI-designated cancer center website, you can search for urologic oncologists who practice at the facility. You can look on the website for biographical information about each of the urologic oncologists to learn about their medical education, training, and experience in treating bladder cancer.

- Ask your friends or acquaintances for recommendations. If you belong to a cancer support group, you can ask for recommendations from other members of the group.

After you have identified a general urologist(s) or urologic oncologist(s), you will want to find out the following:

- Where did the doctor attend medical school and do his or her residency training?
- Is the doctor board certified in urology by the American Board of Medical Specialties (ABMS)? You can find out by clicking on "Is Your Doctor Board Certified?" at *www.certificationmatters.org*.
- How many patients with your form of bladder cancer does the doctor treat each year?
- Have there been any disciplinary actions or malpractice claims brought against the doctor? This information is available from the state medical board in the state where the doctor practices. You can find a directory of state medical boards on the Federation of State Medical Boards' website at *http://www.fsmb.org/policy/contacts*.
- Does the doctor participate in your insurance plan?

If you are looking for a urologic oncologist, you will also want to find out the following:

- Is the doctor fellowship-trained in urologic oncology with expertise in bladder cancer?
- If you are considering a radical cystectomy, you will want to ask how many surgeries of this type the doctor performs each year. What

outcomes, such as complication rates, 5-year-survival rates, and mortality rates, does the surgeon have with respect to this surgery?

- Will the doctor coordinate a multidisciplinary approach to your care if you need to be treated by a medical oncologist and/or a radiation oncologist?

- If you want the option of participating in a clinical trial — are clinical trials available at the hospital where the doctor practices?

You can obtain much of this information by going online to the doctor's office website or hospital website, or by calling the doctor's office. However, it is also very important to meet with the doctor directly. When you first meet the doctor, you will want to get a sense of the doctor's communication style, including whether the doctor answers your questions in a way you can understand. You have to make sure that you are comfortable relating to the doctor. If you live too far away to meet in person, you may be able to talk with the doctor on the telephone or arrange an online consultation. In addition, you may find it helpful, if possible, to talk to a few of the doctor's patients.

TYPES OF ONCOLOGISTS WHO TREAT BLADDER CANCER

Oncology is a branch of medicine that specializes in the diagnosis and treatment of cancer. Within this field, doctors who treat bladder cancer include the following:

- *Urologic oncologists* are urologists who specialize in treating urologic cancers, including bladder cancer, with surgery and other procedures.

- *Medical oncologists* specialize in treating cancer, including bladder cancer, with chemotherapy and immunotherapy.

- *Radiation oncologists* specialize in treating cancer, including bladder cancer, with radiation therapy.

These cancer specialists often work as part of a multidisciplinary team to treat patients with bladder cancer. In most cases, a urologic oncologist will manage the patient's overall care and make referrals, as needed, to a medical oncologist and/or a radiation oncologist.

The information you gather will help you decide which doctor is right for you. Trust your instincts and remember that it may take time for you and your doctor to develop a comfortable relationship. Also remember that if after some time you are not happy with your choice, you can choose a different doctor.

Choosing Your Treatment Facilities

Bladder cancer is a disease that requires specialized treatment, so it is important to find a treatment center that meets your specific needs. The process of finding a hospital or cancer center and choosing a doctor are typically intertwined. Some people first identify a doctor, and then choose a hospital based on where that doctor practices. Others identify a hospital that has a good reputation in treating bladder cancer, and then find a doctor who is on staff at that facility. Chances are you will choose your doctor first, which will determine the hospital or cancer center where you will receive your surgery and/or other cancer treatment. Therefore, before you finalize your decision about which physician to choose, you must be comfortable with the hospital or cancer center where that doctor practices.

The following questions will help you identify the best hospital or cancer center for your particular situation:

- Is the facility one of the 69 National Cancer Institute (NCI)-designated cancer centers?
- How much experience and expertise does the facility have in treating bladder cancer, and how successful has it been with those treatments?
- Does the facility offer the full range of medical services that you will potentially need?
- What cancer support services does the facility offer? Will you have access to oncology social workers, registered dietitians, and other members of an integrated health care team?
- Does the facility offer clinical trials?
- Does the facility accept your insurance?
- Does the facility provide access to cancer-related information and education?

Understanding Your Treatment Options

Once you have full confidence in your diagnosis and have chosen a general urologist or urologic oncologist to manage your treatment and care, the next step is to fully understand your treatment options. Treatment options vary significantly, depending on the diagnosis. Generally, the higher the stage of the disease, the more complex the treatment options.

To gain an understanding of your treatment options, it is important to ask your doctor the following questions:

- What are my treatment options, and what is the treatment goal(s) for each option?
- What are the benefits of each treatment option, and how will the outcome(s) be measured?
- What are the potential short-term and long-term side effects and complications associated with each treatment option? What steps can be taken to minimize and/or prevent them?
- What are the possible late effects of treatment (side effects that appear months or years after treatment ends), if any, associated with each treatment option?
- How will my life be impacted by each treatment option? What will the impact be on my family life and/or work life?
- What is the timeline for each treatment option?
- Who will be administering each treatment option, and where will it be administered (outpatient or inpatient)?
- Should I be considering clinical trials? If so, how do I find clinical trials that are appropriate for my disease?
- What treatment plan do you recommend, and why?

Once you have a full understanding of your treatment options, you will be in a good position to choose a treatment that is right for you. It is important that you have a clear plan of action. Be sure to ask your doctor for a detailed treatment plan, including what will happen, when, and by whom. In addition to communicating with your doctor, you may also need to clarify your medical insurance coverage, arrange for transportation to treatments, or make adjustments to your work schedule or family responsibilities. It is important to reach out to your family, your friends, and your medical team to get the information and support you need to address the full range of medical, social, and emotional needs that often accompany a cancer diagnosis.

Preparing for Your Doctor's Appointments

There are things you can do to prepare for your doctor's appointments that will facilitate effective communication. It is helpful to think in advance about what you want to achieve from your visit and what your doctor needs from you to provide you with the best possible care.

The following are what you need to bring to your appointment, whether it is your first or a subsequent appointment, and whenever you are seeking a second opinion:

- Copies of all relevant medical records. It is important that you ask your doctor what medical records, pathology slides, and/or imaging scans he or she wants you to bring to the appointment or send in advance of your visit. If you send your records, it is a good idea to bring extra copies with you.
- A written list of questions and concerns you want to discuss with your doctor.
- A list of your symptoms (if any), including when they began, their frequency, and how long they last.
- A list of all your medications, including the dosages and how often you take them. This should include prescription drugs and non-prescription, over-the-counter medications, as well as dietary supplements, such as vitamins and herbs.
- Your personal medical history, including any allergies or adverse reactions to medications, as well as your family medical history.
- A pen and notebook or laptop, so you can take notes.
- A recording device to record the meeting, so you can review your conversation. (First ask your doctor for permission to record the consultation.)

- A family member or friend to be a second set of ears — someone who will listen carefully and take notes, and who can help you absorb the information from your visit.

Before leaving the doctor's office, make sure you are clear about the next step(s) of your care, and who to contact if you have further questions.

Careful preparation for your doctor's appointment is important to make your doctor's visit as efficient and productive as possible. Planning ahead will help you address — during the limited time of your doctor's visit — all of the issues that are on your mind.

After your doctor's appointment, it is often helpful to review your notes, notes taken by family members or friends who accompanied you, and/or your recording of the meeting. This gives you an opportunity to reflect on your conversation with your doctor while it is still fresh in your mind. Did your doctor answer all of your questions, and did you understand the answers? Did your doctor mention things that raised additional questions? The process of educating yourself about your disease is ongoing and sometimes confusing. It is important that you continue asking questions until you are satisfied that you fully understand your situation.

Using the Internet

The Internet can be very helpful for people who are seeking information about their type of cancer, or those who are making decisions about their treatment. However, it is important to consider the credibility of the organization that is posting the information, since not all information on the Internet is accurate. Like cancer information found in books, magazines, or newspaper articles, information on the Internet should be used for informational purposes only and is not a substitute for doctors' advice or treatment recommendations. Do not make any changes in your care without first talking with your doctor.

Appendix C, "Bladder Cancer Resources," lists websites that offer educational materials, support, and advocacy for people with bladder cancer and their families and friends.

Keeping Records of Your Bladder Cancer History

Keeping accurate records of your bladder cancer history from the date of your diagnosis is an important part of managing your health care.

There are several reasons to keep your own medical records:

- In some instances, each facility or doctor involved in your care will keep separate medical records of your doctor's visits, diagnostic tests, and treatments. Keeping your own medical records combines these separate records into a complete, unified, collection of medical records, which you are able to store in one place.
- Your personal medical history will always be available to you or a family member when you need it. This is especially important if you are being treated by multiple doctors, receive care at multiple facilities, or transfer to a new doctor or facility. It is also important that you have your own set of records in case your doctor's medical records are ever lost or destroyed or become difficult to obtain because your doctor has relocated or retired.
- By keeping your own set of medical records, you can review the information at your convenience and share it with family members and friends who are supporting you during your cancer journey. With this knowledge, you will feel more in control of your disease and better equipped to participate in treatment decisions.
- Access to your medical records can help you better manage health insurance claims, taxes, and other legal matters, such as disability insurance and life insurance.

Under the federal Health Insurance Portability and Accountability Act of 1996 (HIPAA), you have the right to get copies of your medical records from your health care providers. Most health care providers require that you make a written request on forms that you can obtain from their offices. For more information, go to *www.hhs.gov/ocr/privacy.*

A complete medical history of your bladder cancer diagnosis and treatment should include the following information:

- The date of your diagnosis.
- Detailed information about your diagnosis, including the cell type(s), stage and grade, and number, size, and location of tumor(s).
- Detailed records of all your diagnostic tests and test results, including copies of all surgical, imaging, pathology, and urine cytology reports.
- Detailed records of all your treatments, including surgical procedures, intravesical drug therapy, systemic chemotherapy, and/or radiation therapy. These records should include the dates and descriptions of all treatments — including agents used, treatment regimens, dosages, response to treatment, and related side effects or complications. If you participated in a clinical trial, your records should also include the identifying number and title of the clinical trial.
- Names and contact information of all health care providers and facilities involved in your cancer care.

It is important to keep your records up-to-date, including records of your follow-up doctor's visits and the results of all tests and procedures.

NEXT STEPS

The next steps are to read chapters 3–5 of this book, which provide information all patients need to know to understand their bladder cancer diagnosis. You may then choose to read only the remaining chapter or chapters that apply to your specific diagnosis. Chapter 6 is for patients with *non-muscle-invasive* bladder cancer; chapters 7–12 are for patients with *muscle-invasive* bladder cancer; and chapter 13 is for patients with *metastatic* bladder cancer.

We hope that the information in this book will help you become an informed, proactive patient, with the knowledge and skills to achieve the best possible outcomes for your disease.

CHAPTER 3

An Introduction to the Urinary System

This chapter focuses on the bladder and the larger system of which it is a part — the **urinary system**, also called the **urinary tract**. This chapter also discusses other parts of the anatomy that can be affected by bladder cancer and/or its treatment.

The Urinary System

The organs and other structures that make up the urinary system include the kidneys and ureters (located in the *upper urinary tract*) and the bladder and urethra (located in the *lower urinary tract*). The male and female urinary systems are shown in figures 3.1, 3.2, 3.3, and 3.4.

It is the function of the urinary system to filter out waste products from the blood and dispose of the waste in the form of urine, which ultimately is eliminated from the body. To envision this process, it may be useful to think of the urinary system in terms of water running downhill. The **kidneys**, which filter the blood and produce urine, sit at the top of the urinary tract. From the kidneys, urine travels down two thin tubes, called **ureters**, which transport urine from the kidneys to the **bladder**. The bladder, a hollow, balloon-shaped organ, stores the urine. From the bladder, urine exits the body through a thin tube, called the **urethra**. These organs and structures work together to produce, store, and eliminate urine from the body.

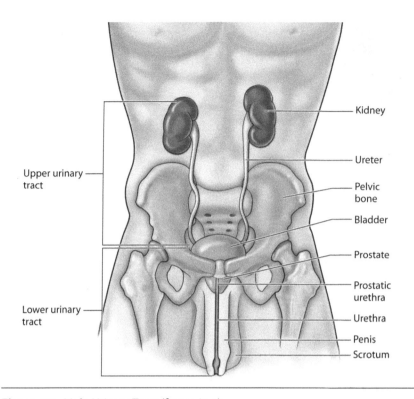

Figure 3.1 Male Urinary Tract (front view)

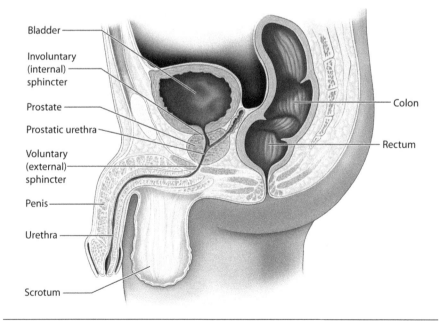

Figure 3.2 Male Lower Urinary Tract (side view)

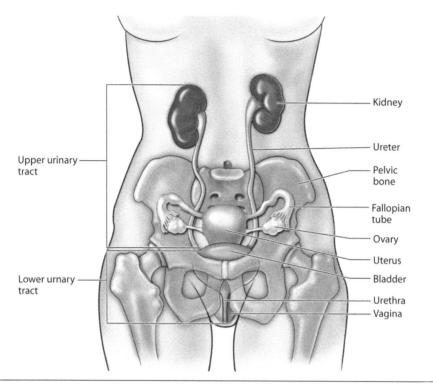

Figure 3.3 Female Urinary Tract (front view)

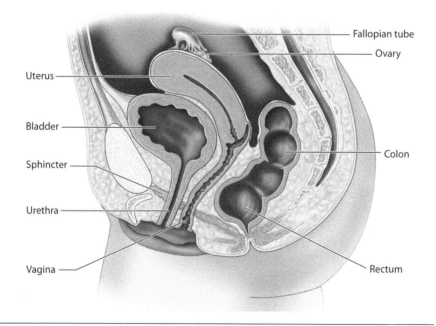

Figure 3.4 Female Lower Urinary Tract (side view)

Kidneys

The *kidneys* are a pair of bean-shaped organs located near the middle of the back, just below the rib cage (see figure 3.5). Each kidney is about 4 to 6 inches

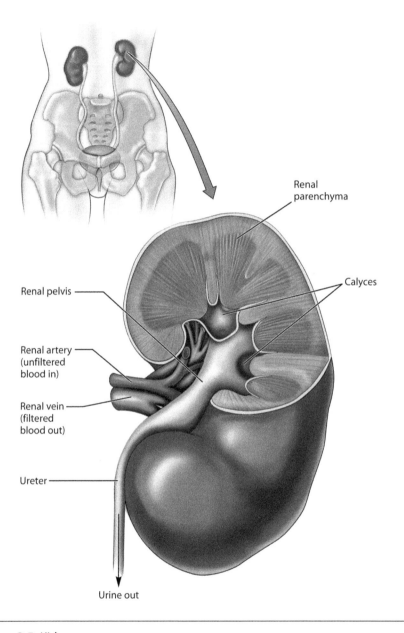

Figure 3.5 Kidneys

long, 2 to 3 inches wide, and 1 to 2 inches thick. Every day, the kidneys filter out about 2 quarts of waste products and extra fluid from the blood and dispose of this waste in the form of urine. This process involves the renal parenchyma, calyces, and renal pelvis, which are located inside each of the kidneys. The *renal parenchyma* filters out waste products and excess fluid from the blood and creates urine, which flows into small, cup-like dividers, called *calyces*, which then channel urine into the *renal pelvis*. The renal pelvis acts as a funnel into the ureters.

Ureters

From the kidneys, urine travels down 2 thin tubes, called **ureters**, to the bladder. Each ureter is about 10 to 12 inches long. Muscles in the ureter walls tighten and relax to push urine downward from the kidneys to the bladder. Each kidney has its own ureter, which attaches to the bladder.

Bladder

The **bladder** is a hollow, balloon-shaped organ situated behind the pelvic bones, surrounded by several organs. In men, the bladder is located just above the prostate and in front of the rectum (see figure 3.2). In women, the bladder is located in front of the vagina and below the uterus, ovaries, and fallopian tubes (see figure 3.4). The triangle-shaped area where the ureters connect to the bladder is called the *trigone*. The walls on either side of the trigone are called the *right* and *left lateral walls*, and the back wall is called the *posterior wall*. The roof of the bladder is called the *dome* (see figures 3.6 and 3.7).

The bladder stores urine, the liquid waste produced by the kidneys. As a store-house for urine, the bladder is constantly filling up and emptying. The bladder expands when urine fills the bladder and contracts when urine exits the bladder. As the bladder fills up, nerves in the bladder create the sensation of having to urinate, and then stimulate the bladder to contract so it can empty. The contraction produces squeezing, which leads to the emptying of urine through the urethra. Although a normal bladder can hold about a pint of urine, it is common for people to experience the urge to urinate when the bladder is about half full.

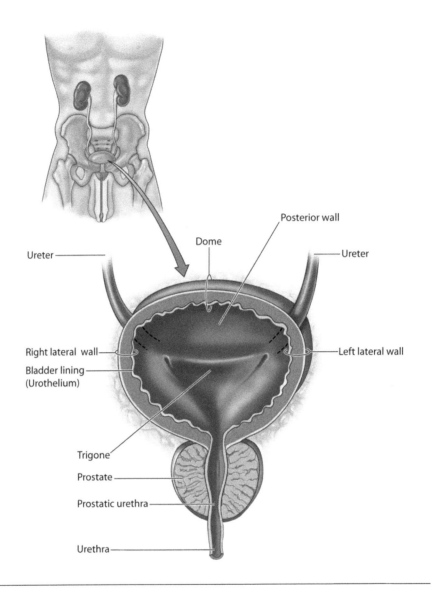

Figure 3.6 Male Bladder

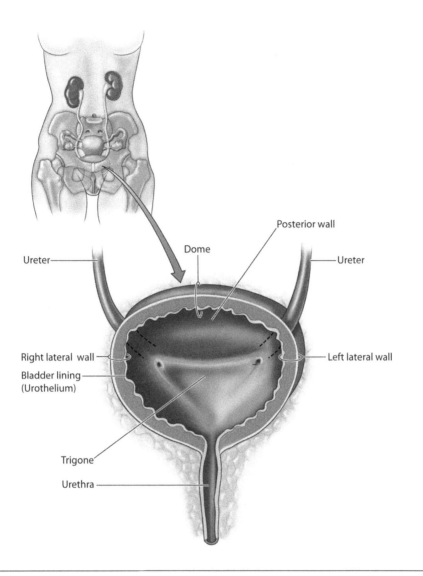

Figure 3.7 Female Bladder

Layers of the Bladder Wall

The bladder has a thick wall composed of several layers, called the **bladder wall** (see figure 3.8). The innermost layer of the bladder wall is referred to as the **bladder lining**, also called the **urothelium**. Other names for the urothelium are *mucosa* and *transitional epithelium*. The next layer of the bladder wall is the **lamina propria**, also called the *submucosa*. The lamina propria is a specialized layer of blood vessels and cells that separate the urothelium from the muscle.

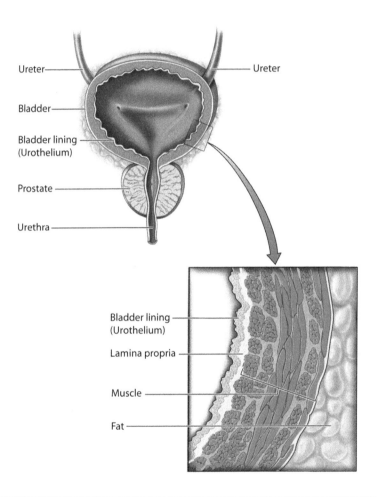

Figure 3.8 Layers of the Bladder Wall

The outermost layer of the bladder wall is the **muscle**, also called the *muscularis propria*, which is composed of thick, smooth, muscle bundles. Around the muscle is a layer of **fat**, also called *perivesical fat*, which separates the muscle from surrounding organs and tissues.

Bladder cancer begins in the bladder lining (urothelium) and, if left unchecked, can invade the lamina propria, muscle, and fat layers. When evaluating your disease, your doctor must determine if there is bladder cancer in one or more of the layers of the bladder wall.

Urethra

The bladder empties into a tube, called the **urethra**, which carries urine from the bladder to outside the body. The structure of the urethra differs somewhat in men and women. In women, the urethra is about 1½ to 2 inches long and exits the body just above the vaginal opening (see figure 3.4). In men, the urethra is about 8 inches long, travels through the prostate and penile shaft, and exits the body through the opening at the end of the penis (see figure 3.2). The portion of the male urethra that runs from the bladder through the prostate is called the *prostatic urethra.*

CANCERS OF THE URINARY TRACT

About 90% of bladder cancer diagnosed in the United States is **urothelial cell carcinoma**, also called **urothelial bladder cancer**. Urothelial bladder cancer begins in the urothelial cells of the bladder lining (urothelium). (The remaining 10% of bladder cancer begins in other cell types in the bladder lining.) It is important to understand that the kidneys, ureters, and urethra are also lined with urothelial cells. When cancer develops in the urothelial cells of the bladder, there is a risk of cancer developing in the urothelial cells of the kidneys, ureters, and/or urethra, as well. Therefore, when diagnosing bladder cancer, doctors must evaluate all areas of the urinary system.

The Prostate, Urinary Sphincters, and Lymph Nodes

Other parts of the body that may be affected by bladder cancer and/or its treatment include the prostate, the urinary sphincters, and the lymph nodes.

Prostate

The **prostate** is a walnut-sized gland located below the bladder in men (see figure 3.6). Women do not have a prostate. The prostate produces seminal fluid, the liquid that contains the sperm during the process of ejaculation. The prostate is always removed when a male patient has surgery to remove the bladder, called a *radical cystectomy*. The removal of the prostate during a radical cystectomy may have unwanted consequences for the male patient. Prostate removal is associated with changes related to sexual function, fertility, and continence.

Urinary Sphincters

The **urinary sphincters** are responsible for urinary control, known as *continence*. Both men and women have two urinary sphincters, an *involuntary* (internal) sphincter and a *voluntary* (external) sphincter. Sphincters are circular, donut-shaped muscles surrounding the urethra. When either the involuntary or the voluntary sphincter contracts, it constricts the urethra and prevents urine from leaking.

In men, urinary control is maintained through the complex interaction of the two sphincters, with the involuntary (internal) sphincter the primary control mechanism (see figure 3.2). The involuntary sphincter is located at the junction of the bladder and the prostate. The voluntary (external) sphincter is located just below the prostate. When the prostate is removed during a radical cystectomy, the patient loses the involuntary sphincter. Consequently, the male patient must thereafter rely on the voluntary sphincter for urinary control.

In women, the function of the urinary sphincters and the mechanism of urinary control are much less well understood than in men. The current medical thinking is that both voluntary and involuntary sphincters exist in women just as they do in men — but the precise anatomic locations of the involuntary and voluntary control muscles that make up the female sphincters are difficult to identify. Nonetheless, the female sphincter apparatus is a robust control mechanism that performs all of the same duties as its male counterpart.

Lymph Nodes

Lymph nodes are rounded masses of tissue, about the same size and shape as baked beans, scattered throughout the body, including near the bladder (see figure 3.9).

Lymph nodes are part of the *lymphatic system,* which plays a major role in the body's immune system — the mechanism in the body that fights disease. The lymphatic system is composed of a series of interconnecting channels, called *lymphatic vessels,* which serve as a "highway" for cells to travel through the tissues

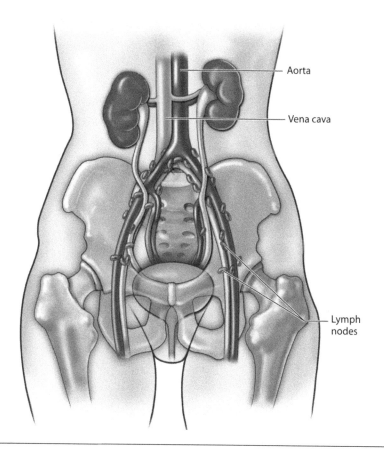

Figure 3.9 Lymph Nodes

31

of the body. The immune cells (various types of white blood cells) that inhabit the lymphatic system continuously survey the body for signs of infection and cancer. Lymph nodes act as weigh stations on the lymphatic highway where the immune cells gather to detect and fight various forms of disease.

Unfortunately, diseases like cancer use the lymphatic highway for their own destructive purposes. Certain types of cancer, including bladder cancer, use the lymphatic vessels to spread from the original site of the cancer (in this case, the bladder) to nearby lymph nodes and distant parts of the body.

Because lymph nodes are often the first sites affected by the spread of cancer outside the bladder, lymph nodes are surgically removed during a radical cystectomy to determine if the disease has spread to the lymph nodes. If bladder cancer is found in the lymph nodes, there is a high risk the disease will metastasize (spread), or has already metastasized, to distant sites in the body.

CHAPTER 4

Diagnosing Bladder Cancer: Procedures and Tests

Doctors use various tools and techniques to diagnose bladder cancer. A comprehensive evaluation of this disease includes some or all of the following procedures and tests (discussed in detail later in this chapter).

Cystoscopy: A cystoscopy is a diagnostic procedure used to visually examine the lining of the bladder to see if abnormal tissue is present. If during the procedure, the doctor sees suspicious-looking tissue, a small sample of tissue, called a *biopsy*, can be removed from the bladder lining (urothelium). The biopsy is sent to a pathology laboratory for examination under a microscope to determine if cancer is present. A cystoscopy is a minimally invasive procedure performed under local anesthesia in the doctor's office. Although a cystoscopy is an important diagnostic tool, it does not, by itself, provide a complete diagnosis of bladder cancer. Thus, a cystoscopy is usually performed in conjunction with other diagnostic tests and procedures, such as urine tests, imaging tests, a TURBT, and/or a blue light cystoscopy.

Urine tests: Urine tests can detect changes in urine cells that indicate the presence of cancer in the bladder or other parts of the urinary tract. Sometimes cancer can be detected in urine cells before abnormal tissue can be detected visually during a cystoscopy or TURBT. The oldest and most common urine test is *urine cytology,* which is routinely performed to evaluate patients with bladder cancer.

Imaging tests: Imaging tests are used to detect bladder cancer that has spread outside the bladder to lymph nodes, surrounding organs, and/or distant sites in the body, such as the liver, lung, or bone. Imaging tests are also used to detect tumors in the urinary tract, especially the upper urinary tract (kidneys and ureters). The types of imaging tests discussed in this chapter are a CT (computed tomography) scan, a CT urogram, an MRI (magnetic resonance imaging) scan, a PET-CT scan, and an ultrasound.

TURBT: When it is suspected or determined that a patient has bladder cancer based on a prior cystoscopy, urine test, or imaging test, the next step is usually a procedure called a *TURBT*. **TURBT** stands for **T**rans**U**rethral **R**esection of **B**ladder **T**umor. A TURBT is similar to a cystoscopy — in that a TURBT allows the doctor to visually examine the bladder lining. However, a TURBT allows the doctor to obtain more extensive biopsies than with a cystoscopy — and to remove tumors from the bladder wall. Because a TURBT is a more invasive procedure than a cystoscopy, it is performed under general anesthesia in an outpatient surgical center or hospital. All biopsies and/or tumors removed during a TURBT are sent to a pathology laboratory for examination under a microscope to determine if cancer is present.

Blue light cystoscopy: A blue light cystoscopy is a relatively new procedure that is increasingly being used to better diagnose patients with suspected or known tumors in the bladder lining. A blue light cystoscopy is similar to a TURBT — but blue light cystoscopy incorporates the use of an imaging solution and blue light to improve the visualization of tumors. Like a TURBT, a blue light cystoscopy is performed under general anesthesia in an outpatient surgical center or hospital.

The remainder of this chapter discusses in more detail the use of cystoscopy, urine tests, imaging tests, TURBT, and blue light cystoscopy to diagnose bladder cancer.

COMMON SYMPTOMS OF BLADDER CANCER

Most people diagnosed with bladder cancer experience one or more symptoms of the disease. The most common symptom of bladder cancer is **hematuria**, a condition in which there is blood in the urine. Hematuria can be either gross or microscopic. *Gross* means the blood is visible to the naked eye, whereas *microscopic* means the blood is visible only under a microscope. The risk of having bladder cancer is about 3 times higher with gross hematuria than with microscopic hematuria.

If you see blood in your urine (gross hematuria), be sure to report this symptom to your doctor. Microscopic hematuria is usually detected in a urine sample taken during a routine physical examination. Because gross hematuria can occur intermittently, and usually occurs without other symptoms, many patients tend to ignore this symptom. You should always tell your doctor if you see blood in your urine, even if you see it only once. Other possible symptoms of bladder cancer include irritation or pain during urination, frequent urination, and/or an urgent need to urinate. Having one or more of these symptoms does not necessarily mean you have bladder cancer.

Most doctors who evaluate hematuria or other symptoms of bladder cancer start by performing two laboratory tests — a urinalysis and a urine culture — to determine if there is a urinary tract infection, which is often the cause of the symptoms. Other causes of the symptoms include benign conditions, such as kidney stones, or blood-thinning medications. If based on these tests, you do not have a urinary tract infection and there is no other explanation for your symptoms, you should be evaluated for bladder cancer by a *urologist*, a doctor who specializes in treating diseases of the urinary tract.

If you have symptoms of bladder cancer, they should be evaluated promptly. For patients with bladder cancer that is detected and treated early, the prognosis (likely disease outcome) is usually excellent.

Cystoscopy

A *cystoscopy* is one of the first diagnostic procedures for diagnosing bladder cancer. During this procedure, the doctor visually examines the lining of the bladder, using an instrument called a *cystoscope* (see figure 4.1). A cystoscope is a thin, lighted, flexible tube, equipped with a series of fiber optic lenses that allow focused and wide-angle views of the bladder lining using white light. Flexible cystoscopes are made of plastic so they can bend to conform to the contours of the curving path of the urethra.

During a cystoscopy, a cystoscope is passed through the urethra into the bladder. Although this is an invasive procedure, it is minimally so. For men, because of the longer male urethra, a cystoscopy can produce some discomfort. In men, the prostate wraps around a portion of the urethra called the *prostatic urethra*. If the prostate is enlarged or inflamed, this can narrow the urethra and give the doctor less room to maneuver. A flexible cystoscope makes inserting the cystoscope into the urethra easier and produces fewer irritative symptoms. Women tend to tolerate the procedure better than men. This is partly because of the female anatomy and partly because women are more familiar with pelvic

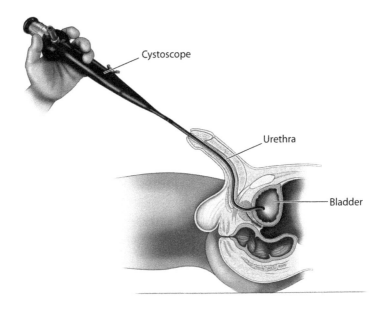

Figure 4.1 Cystoscopy

examinations in general. In fact, most women who undergo a cystoscopy report that the procedure is less uncomfortable than a pelvic exam.

A cystoscopy is usually performed under local anesthesia in the doctor's office and generally takes about 3 to 5 minutes. In preparation for this procedure, you will be given an antiseptic wash around your urethra and surrounding structures, followed by an application of a medicated gel packed with a local anesthetic, called *lidocaine*, to numb the inside of your urethra. During the cystoscopy, your doctor is able to see your bladder lining either directly through the lens of the cystoscope or on a television screen. A tiny camera inside the cystoscope allows your doctor to record any abnormal findings. During the procedure, your bladder will be inflated with fluid and then deflated, during which you will feel a sensation of filling and emptying. This is done to smooth out the bladder's normal folds and wrinkles, so your doctor can get a good look at the interior of the bladder walls.

If during the cystoscopy your doctor sees suspicious-looking tissue, he or she may obtain a small sample of tissue (biopsy) from the bladder lining. If the doctor thinks a small biopsy will not be sufficient to evaluate your bladder, or if a tumor(s) is seen during the cystoscopy, your doctor will need to perform a TURBT to obtain additional biopsies and/or remove the tumors. Any tissue removed during a cystoscopy is sent to a pathology laboratory to be examined by a *pathologist*, a doctor who specializes in identifying cancer by examining cells and tissues under a microscope. Based on this examination, the pathologist records his or her findings in a *pathology report*, which indicates if cancer is present.

After undergoing a cystoscopy, you may experience stinging and burning during urination for a day or two. Blood in the urine, particularly right after the procedure, is common and is not an immediate cause for alarm. Your doctor may prescribe an antibiotic for a few days to lower the risk of developing a urinary tract infection from the procedure.

Although a cystoscopy is an important diagnostic tool, it does not, by itself, provide a complete diagnosis of bladder cancer. Thus, this procedure is usually performed in conjunction with other diagnostic tests and procedures, such as urine tests, imaging tests, a TURBT, and/or a blue light cystoscopy.

Urine Tests

Doctors usually use one or more urine tests, such as the following, when evaluating patients for bladder cancer.

Urine Cytology

The oldest and most common urine test is **urine cytology**. It is routinely used to evaluate patients for bladder cancer.

The bladder lining continually sheds cells that collect in urine. Urine cytology involves the microscopic examination of cells shed from the bladder lining to determine if cancer is present. A sample can be taken from urine collected in the doctor's office, called *voided* urine, or from urine drained from the bladder during a cystoscopy or TURBT, called a *bladder wash*. Because cells from other areas of the urinary tract (urethra, kidneys, and ureters) also shed into urine, a finding of cancer cells in a urine sample may indicate cancer in other areas of the urinary tract, as well.

A *cytopathologist* is a doctor who specializes in analyzing cells found in body fluids, such as urine. A cytopathologist examines cells from a urine sample under a microscope to determine if cancer is present. This is called *urine cytology*. The cytopathologist writes a cytology report, which indicates if the cells in the urine sample are *benign* (noncancerous), *malignant* (cancerous), or *atypical* (suspicious for cancer) — and, if cancerous, whether the cells are *low grade* (not aggressive) or *high grade* (aggressive). A finding of low-grade and/or high-grade cancer cells in the urine requires further evaluation, even when a cystoscopy appears normal. A finding of *atypical* cells in the urine, although not definitive, also requires further evaluation, because of the possibility that cancer may be present in the bladder or elsewhere in the urinary tract but has not yet been detected.

Studies have shown that urine cytology has a detection rate of less than 50% for *low-grade* bladder cancer — compared to a detection rate of 95% to 100% for *high-grade* bladder cancer. Although urine cytology is not very accurate in detecting low-grade disease, it is a very useful and important tool in detecting high-grade disease.

Sometimes urine cytology detects cancer before it is visible during a cystoscopy or TURBT. Urine cytology is especially helpful in detecting a form of high-grade bladder cancer, called **CIS** (**C**arcinoma **I**n **S**itu), which can be difficult to see during a cystoscopy or TURBT.

There can be a range of interpretations of urine cytology among cytopathologists, so the findings of urine cytology are subjective to a certain extent. It may be reassuring to get a second opinion from a second cytopathologist to confirm your initial diagnosis.

Other Urine Tests

Although urine cytology is the oldest and most commonly used urine test for diagnosing bladder cancer, other urine tests have been developed over the last 20 years that are slowly being incorporated into practice. These tests look for specific molecular and genetic markers that are released by bladder cancer cells. These tests include BTA, NMP22, FISH (UroVysion), and Immunocyt. Generally speaking, these tests are used in conjunction with urine cytology. However, urine tests should never be used alone to make a bladder cancer diagnosis.

Imaging Tests

Imaging tests are used to detect bladder cancer that has spread outside the bladder to lymph nodes, surrounding organs, and/or distant sites in the body, such as the liver, lung, or bone. Imaging tests are also used to detect tumors in the urinary tract, especially the upper urinary tract (kidneys and ureters) — which are not examined during a cystoscopy or TURBT. The imaging tests discussed in this chapter are non-invasive, which means they are performed without entering the body.

There are advantages and disadvantages of each type of imaging test. Which test(s) your doctor recommends will depend on a number of factors, including your medical history, the reason(s) for ordering the test(s), and your doctor's and your personal preferences.

CT Scan

A *CT (computed tomography) scan* is used to evaluate areas outside the bladder to determine if cancer is present. A CT scan can detect the spread of bladder cancer to lymph nodes, surrounding organs, and distant sites in the body. A CT scan provides detailed images by taking a series of X-rays from various angles and reconstructing them into three-dimensional images.

Prior to undergoing a CT scan, you will be given instructions on how to prepare for the test. Most doctors recommend not eating or drinking for 8 hours before a CT scan. Although the scan itself takes only about 10 or 15 minutes, you should plan on spending at least an hour at your appointment because of the time it takes to answer questions about your medical history and be prepared for the test.

A CT scanner is a large, donut-shaped machine linked to a computer. During the test, you will lie on your back on a table that is attached to the scanner. You will be moved in and out of the scanner as the machine takes digital pictures of your body. While the images are being taken, you will be asked to hold your breath and remain still for short periods of time, because bodily movement can blur the images. The imaging data is fed into a computer, which transforms the data into a series of images.

Contrast dyes are often used to improve the quality of images produced by the scan. You will likely receive contrast dyes both orally (by mouth) and intravenously (by injection into a vein). Before the test begins, you will be asked to drink a few glasses of a liquid contrast dye containing either iodine or barium. In addition, an IV (intravenous) line will be inserted into a vein in your hand or arm. Then, part way through the test, contrast dye containing iodine will be injected through the IV line. The intravenous contrast dye usually creates a warm, flushed feeling throughout the body but is well tolerated by most patients. Those patients allergic to shellfish and/or iodine-based contrast dyes are better served by an MRI, which does not use an iodine-based contrast dye.

Patients often ask about the safety of CT scans because of concerns about overexposure to radiation. Most contemporary studies indicate that modern diagnostic imaging tests do not significantly increase the risk of developing cancer as a result of exposure to radiation during the test. If you have questions about the number of scans your doctor is ordering, you should discuss your concerns with your doctor.

The advantages of a CT scan are that it provides very detailed, high-quality images, and is relatively quick and easy to tolerate. The disadvantages are exposure to radiation and the risk of an allergic reaction to an iodine-based contrast dye.

CT Urogram

You may hear the term ***CT urogram*** (CTU) and wonder how it differs from a CT scan. A CT urogram is a specialized CT scan, which provides more detailed images of the urinary tract than those produced by a conventional CT scan. Whereas a CT scan is typically used to look for bladder cancer that has spread outside the urinary tract, a CT urogram is more commonly used when it is thought that the cancer is confined to the bladder and/or other areas of the urinary tract.

MRI

MRI (magnetic resonance imaging) produces detailed images similar to a CT scan, but it uses radio waves and powerful magnets instead of radiation. Like a CT scan, an MRI is used to look at areas outside the bladder to detect the spread of bladder cancer to lymph nodes, surrounding organs, and/or distant parts of the body.

Generally, there are no special restrictions on what you can eat or drink before an MRI. If you have a history of impaired kidney function, you may need a blood test to determine if you have sufficient kidney function to safely have an MRI with contrast dye. Although the MRI itself takes about 30 to 45 minutes, you should plan on spending at least 90 minutes at your appointment to allow time to answer questions and to be prepared for the test. Before the test, you will be asked questions about your medical history, including whether you have any metal devices inside your body. Anyone with a metal device implanted inside his or her body cannot safely undergo an MRI. You will also be asked to remove all metal objects from your body, including jewelry, dentures, and glasses.

An MRI scanner is a narrow, tunnel-shaped tube, which is actually an array of very powerful magnets. When undergoing an MRI, you will lie on a table that slides inside an MRI scanner. An MRI technologist will place pads on your body and advance you into the scanner. Patients who have claustrophobia (a fear of small, confined spaces) may find this aspect of the test uncomfortable. If you have a problem with claustrophobia, you should discuss this with your doctor ahead of time. You may be able to take a mild sedative to relax you during the test.

While inside the MRI scanner, you will hear loud, banging noises when the machine begins to take pictures. Because of the loud noises inside the scanner, you will wear earplugs and/or headphones during the test. If the MRI technologist does not give you earplugs and/or headphones, you should ask for them. During the test, you can speak with the MRI technologist through a microphone to ask questions or discuss any problems you are experiencing.

If you are having intravenous contrast dye with your MRI, an IV (intravenous) line will be inserted into a vein in your hand or arm prior to the test. The contrast dye used with an MRI is not iodine-based as it is with a CT scan, so an MRI can be performed safely on patients allergic to iodine-based dyes. However, the contrast dye used with an MRI, called *gadolinium*, can be harmful to people with certain medical conditions, such as impaired kidney function. If you have kidney disease, you can have an MRI without contrast dye.

The advantages of an MRI are that it provides very detailed, high-quality images; there is no exposure to radiation; and patients allergic to iodine-based contrast dye can have the test. The disadvantages are that some patients experience discomfort due to claustrophobia and/or the length of the test, and that patients who have metal devices inside their body cannot safely have an MRI.

PET-CT

In certain circumstances, the findings of a CT scan or MRI can be ambiguous, leaving doctors unable to discern whether an abnormality is related to cancer or to some potentially benign process. A newer type of imaging scan that combines PET (positron emission tomography) and CT (computed tomography) technologies, called a **PET-CT** scan, permits physicians to address this difficult situation.

PET technology is based on the observation that normal cells and cancer cells digest (metabolize) sugar at different rates. Before undergoing a PET-CT scan, you will be given a small amount of radioactive material (called *tracer*) containing sugar, which is administered intravenously. The tracer travels through the blood and collects in organs and tissues. The tracer is metabolized by normal tissue and cancerous tissue at different rates, which the PET-CT scan can detect and record.

The combination of PET and CT technologies provides information that enables doctors to determine whether an ambiguous finding on a conventional CT scan or an MRI suggests the presence of cancer.

Ultrasound

An **ultrasound** is often used as an initial imaging test to evaluate the bladder and kidneys. The test works by using sound waves that bounce off internal organs. This creates images of the urinary tract that can show tumors, blockages, blood clots, and kidney stones.

Since sound waves travel best through fluid, you may be asked to drink fluids prior to the test to fill your bladder. You will be lying on a table during the test, which usually takes about 20 to 30 minutes.

The advantages of an ultrasound are that it is painless, does not use radiation, and is very safe — with no known side effects or adverse reactions. The disadvantages are that images produced lack fine detail, and small tumors can be missed. In addition, an ultrasound cannot detect cancer in the ureters. Consequently, additional imaging tests, such as a CT scan, a CT urogram, or an MRI, may be needed.

TURBT

A *TURBT* (also called a **TUR**, which stands for **T**rans**U**rethral **R**esection) is similar to a cystoscopy in that a lighted tube is passed through the urethra into the bladder (see figure 4.2). However, instead of a cystoscope, the urologist uses an instrument called a *resectoscope*, which is rigid and larger than a cystoscope. A resectoscope is equipped with a camera, a wide-angle telescope, and channels

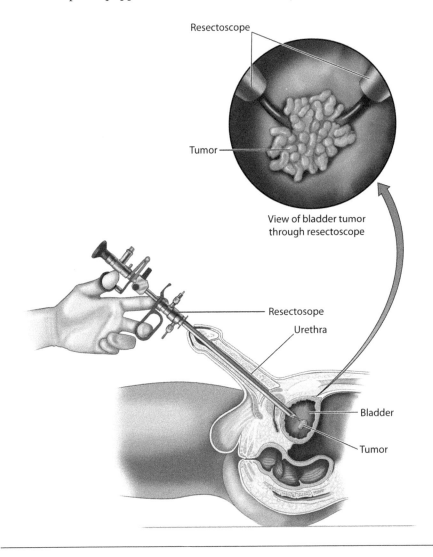

Resectoscope

Tumor

View of bladder tumor through resectoscope

Resectosope

Urethra

Bladder

Tumor

4.2 TURBT

that permit the passage of special tools into the bladder. During a TURBT, the doctor is able to see the lining of the bladder either directly through the lens of the resectoscope or on a television screen. A resectoscope allows the doctor to obtain tissue samples (biopsies) that cannot be obtained during a cystoscopy — and to remove entire tumors.

A TURBT is performed under general anesthesia in an outpatient surgical center or hospital. Your doctor will advise you about how to prepare for a TURBT — including when to stop eating and drinking and which medications to stop taking prior to the procedure — and what to expect during your recovery.

During a TURBT, your doctor may take *random biopsies* (random samples of tissue that appear normal) to check for hidden disease. Random biopsies are useful for detecting tumors too small to be seen during a cystoscopy or TURBT. Taking random biopsies may be especially helpful when urine cytology indicates cancer, but no abnormalities are seen during a cystoscopy or TURBT.

A TURBT can be performed for both diagnostic and treatment purposes. Obtaining biopsies to determine if cancer is present is a diagnostic use of a TURBT, whereas removing tumors is a treatment use of a TURBT. The uses of a TURBT for treating bladder cancer are discussed in chapters 6 and 12.

It is not unusual for a doctor to use a TURBT for treatment and diagnostic purposes during the same procedure. For example, at the same time that the doctor removes a bladder tumor (a treatment use), he or she might also obtain biopsies to check for additional disease (a diagnostic use).

All biopsies and/or tumors removed during a TURBT are sent to a pathology laboratory to be examined under a microscope by a pathologist. Although waiting for the results may cause worry, the careful evaluation of tissue removed from the bladder is key to getting a complete and accurate diagnosis. The pathologist will provide your doctor with a pathology report, indicating whether cancer is present and, if so, the nature and extent of the disease.

Blue Light Cystoscopy

A relatively new procedure, called **blue light cystoscopy** (also called *fluorescence cystoscopy*), is increasingly being used to better diagnose patients with suspected or known tumors in the bladder lining. It is important not to confuse a traditional cystoscopy, which uses a flexible tube and is performed under local anesthesia in the doctor's office — with a blue light cystoscopy, which uses a larger, rigid tube and is performed under general anesthesia in an outpatient surgical center or hospital. Blue light cystoscopy is an enhanced imaging procedure that improves the visualization of tumors. This can lead to better detection and more complete removal of tumors.

Blue light cystoscopy was licensed in Europe in 2005 and is widely used today in Europe. In 2010, the Food and Drug Administration (FDA) approved blue light cystoscopy for use in the United States, where its use is increasing.

A TURBT views the bladder under white light alone, whereas a blue light cystoscopy views the bladder under both white light and blue light. A blue light cystoscopy uses an imaging solution, called *Cysview®*. This imaging solution is instilled into the bladder through a catheter at least one hour before the procedure. Cysview® contains fluorescent compounds. These compounds are absorbed by rapidly growing cells, such as cancer cells. When viewed under blue light, the fluorescent compounds that are absorbed by cancer cells appear *red* — allowing better visualization of cancerous tissue, particularly small or indistinct tumors that may be missed when viewed under white light alone. Blue light cystoscopy can lead to more complete detection and more accurate staging — resulting in better treatment decisions and reduced risk of recurrence.

The use of blue light cystoscopy as a diagnostic tool should be considered when patients are suspected or known to have tumors in the bladder lining.

When using Cysview®, fluorescence of non-cancerous cells can occur, resulting in a false-positive diagnosis. The percentage of false-positive diagnoses with blue light cystoscopy is comparable to that with cystoscopy or TURBT using white light alone.

Use of Diagnostic Procedures and Tests After Initial Diagnosis

The results of the procedures and tests discussed in this chapter are the basis for your bladder cancer diagnosis. After your initial diagnosis, these procedures and tests will continue to be used to assess your response to treatment and will be part of a lifelong surveillance program to monitor for recurrence and/or progression of your disease.

CHAPTER 5

Understanding Your Bladder Cancer Diagnosis

Based on the results of your diagnostic procedures and tests, you will get a *diagnosis*, which identifies whether or not you have bladder cancer — and, if so, the aggressiveness (grade), depth and extent (stage), and cell type of your disease. This chapter provides you with information you need to know to understand your diagnosis and have meaningful conversations with your doctor about your treatment options and prognosis (likely outcome of your disease).

If you are diagnosed with bladder cancer, you will need to ask the following questions:

- What is the **grade** of my bladder cancer?
- What is the **stage** of my bladder cancer?
- What is the **cell type** of my bladder cancer?
- What does my bladder cancer **diagnosis** mean?
- What are my risks of **recurrence** and/or **progression**?
- Should I get a **second opinion**?

What Is the Grade of My Bladder Cancer?

The **grade** of bladder cancer indicates the potential of the cancer to be aggressive and do harm. The current grading system classifies bladder cancer cells as **low grade** or **high grade.** Older grading systems assigned a number between 1 and 3 (lowest to highest grade) to bladder cancer cells.

Low-grade cancer cells closely resemble normal cells, tend to grow slowly, and have a low risk of progressing to the deeper layers of the bladder wall and causing harm.

High-grade cancer cells bear little resemblance to normal cells, tend to grow quickly, and have a high risk of progressing to the deeper layers of the bladder wall and/or to other parts of the body.

What Is the Stage of My Bladder Cancer?

The *stage* of bladder cancer indicates the depth of invasion and extent of disease spread (see figure 5.1). Stage answers the questions: How far has the cancer spread? Is it confined to the bladder lining, or has it invaded more deeply into the bladder wall? Has it reached the lamina propria? Has it reached the muscle layer, or penetrated into the fat around the bladder? Has the cancer metastasized (spread) to nearby lymph nodes or distant sites in the body? The farther away the disease has grown from its point of origin in the bladder lining, the higher the stage of the disease, and the more harm it can cause.

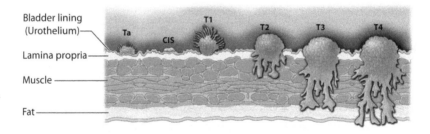

Figure 5.1 Stages of Bladder Cancer

The TNM Staging System

The American Joint Committee on Cancer (AJCC) and the Union Internationale Contre le Cancer (UICC) put forth a system for staging cancer, called the *TNM staging system* (see figure 5.2). This system classifies cancer stages by combining the initials **T** (primary tumor), **N** (lymph node), and **M** (distant metastasis). The initial T indicates the depth and extent of the primary (original) tumor; the initial N indicates the absence or presence of lymph node involvement; and the initial M indicates the absence or presence of distant metastasis.

The TNM Staging System for Bladder Cancer

PRIMARY TUMOR (T)

Ta   Cancer is confined to the bladder lining, called the *urothelium* (mucosa or transitional epithelium).

CIS (TIS)   Carcinoma in situ, a flat tumor confined to the *urothelium.*

T1   Cancer invades the *lamina propria* (submucosa), a specialized layer of blood vessels and cells that separates the urothelium from the muscle.

T2   Cancer invades the *muscle* (muscularis propria).
        T2a: Superficially
        T2b: More deeply

T3   Cancer penetrates through the muscle into the *fat* around the muscle.
        T3a: Microscopically
        T3b: Macroscopically

T4   Cancer invades *certain organs or structures surrounding the bladder.*
        T4a: Invades the prostate in men; invades the vagina or uterus in women.
        T4b: Invades the rectum, pelvic wall, or abdominal wall.

LYMPH NODE (N)

N0   No cancer is present in lymph node(s).

N1   Cancer is present in one lymph node near the bladder.

N2   Cancer is present in more than one lymph node near the bladder.

N3   Cancer is present in lymph nodes located at some distance from the bladder.

DISTANT METASTASIS (M)

M0   There is no evidence of distant metastasis.

M1   There is evidence of distant metastasis.

Figure 5.2 TNM Staging System for Bladder Cancer

According to the TNM staging system, a tumor classified as T1 N0 M0 means the tumor invades the lamina propria (T1), but there is no evidence of lymph node involvement (N0) or distant metastasis (M0). A tumor classified as T2 N1 M0 means the tumor invades the muscle (T2), cancer has spread to one lymph node near the bladder, and there is no evidence of distant metastasis (M0). A tumor classified as T3 N2 M1 means the tumor invades the fat around the muscle (T3), cancer has spread to more than one lymph node near the bladder (N2), and there is evidence of distant metastasis (M1).

What Is the Cell Type of My Bladder Cancer?

All bladder cancer originates in the cells of the bladder lining. The bladder cancer *cell type* is determined by the kind of cell in which the cancer originates. About 90% of bladder cancer diagnosed in the United States originates in the urothelial cells of the bladder lining. This type of bladder cancer is called *urothelial cell carcinoma*, also called *transitional cell carcinoma*.

About 5% of bladder cancer diagnosed in the United States is *squamous cell carcinoma*. The remaining 5% are rare cell types, including *adenocarcinoma*, *small cell carcinoma*, and *sarcoma*, all of which are aggressive forms of the disease.

The words *carcinoma* and *cancer* mean the same thing.

Urothelial Cell Carcinoma

There are different forms of urothelial cell carcinoma. The different forms of the disease are characterized by different patterns of growth and capacity to do harm. These growth patterns include the following:

- *Papillary* tumors look like seaweed or coral on a stem. They tend to grow into the hollow center of the bladder rather than invade the deeper layers of the bladder wall. They are typically low grade and not likely to spread beyond the bladder lining and be aggressive.

- *Sessile* tumors are solid masses. Unlike papillary tumors, sessile tumors can grow through the lining of the bladder into the deeper layers of the bladder wall. They are typically high grade and more aggressive than papillary tumors.

- *Carcinoma in situ* (CIS) are flat tumors, which may appear as a red velvety patch on the bladder lining. CIS is always high grade and tends to be aggressive. CIS has the potential to spread outside of the bladder with little warning — without first invading the muscle layer of the bladder wall.

- *Micropapillary* tumors are a relatively uncommon form of urothelial cell carcinoma. They are always high grade and very aggressive, and should be treated accordingly.

What Does My Bladder Cancer Diagnosis Mean?

Your bladder cancer diagnosis is a combination of many factors, the most important of which are the grade (aggressiveness), stage (depth and extent), and cell type of your bladder cancer. Other factors to be considered are how many tumors you have, the size of the tumor(s), and the location(s) of the tumor(s).

Grade

The first aspect of your diagnosis to focus on is the *grade* (aggressiveness) of your bladder cancer. The *aggressiveness* of your disease indicates how likely it is to progress (grow) to the deeper layers of the bladder wall and spread to other sites in your body. *Low-grade* bladder cancer is significantly less aggressive and less likely to cause harm than *high-grade* bladder cancer. It is rare for low-grade disease to progress to high-grade disease. Low-grade bladder cancer has a much better prognosis than high-grade bladder cancer. Because of these differences, low-grade bladder cancer and high-grade bladder cancer are often thought of as two different diseases, with low-grade disease far less dangerous than high-grade disease.

Stage

The next aspect of your diagnosis to focus on is the *stage* (depth and extent) of your bladder cancer. There are a number of stages of bladder cancer (see figures 5.1 and 5.2). The lower your stage, the better your prognosis.

This book groups the stages of bladder cancer into *non-muscle-invasive* bladder cancer, *muscle-invasive* bladder cancer, and *metastatic* bladder cancer. These groupings are based on how the stages of bladder cancer are treated. Stages treated similarly are grouped in the same category.

- *Non-muscle-invasive bladder cancer* refers to stages *Ta, CIS*, and *T1*. These are the least invasive stages — and in most cases major surgery is not required. Ta is about twice as likely to be low grade as high grade; CIS is always high grade; and T1 is almost always high grade. In some cases, patients have Ta or T1 tumors in combination with CIS. About 75% of people have non-muscle-invasive bladder cancer at the time of diagnosis. For information about non-muscle-invasive bladder cancer and how it is treated, see chapter 6.

- *Muscle-invasive bladder cancer* refers to stages *T2, T3*, and *T4a*. These stages are always high grade, very dangerous, and, in most cases, require major surgery. Once bladder cancer invades the *muscle* of the bladder wall, it is called *muscle-invasive*. Although stage T3 (cancer that invades the fat around the muscle) and stage T4a (cancer that invades the prostate in men and the vagina or uterus in women) extend *beyond* the muscle, they are included in the *muscle-invasive* category because they are treated the same as muscle-invasive bladder cancer. About 20% of people have muscle-invasive bladder cancer at the time of diagnosis. For information about muscle-invasive bladder cancer and how it is treated, see chapters 7–12.

- *Metastatic bladder cancer* refers to stages *N1, N2, N3, M1*, and *T4b*. Stages N1, N2, and N3 have metastasized (spread) to lymph node(s) in the body. M1 has metastasized to distant site(s), such as the liver, lung, or bone. Stage T4b (cancer that invades the rectum, pelvic wall, or abdominal wall) is included in the *metastatic* category because the treatment for stage T4b is the same as for metastatic disease. The primary treatment for metastatic bladder cancer is systemic chemotherapy. It is the most advanced form of bladder cancer and the most difficult to treat. About 5% of bladder cancer is metastatic at the time of diagnosis. For a discussion of metastatic bladder cancer and how it is treated, see chapter 13.

Cell Type

The third aspect of your diagnosis to focus on is the **cell type** of your bladder cancer. If you are one of the 90% of patients with bladder cancer diagnosed with **urothelial cell carcinoma**, you will want to know the growth pattern of your tumor (discussed earlier in this chapter). *Papillary* tumors are usually low grade and least likely to do harm. *Sessile* (solid) tumors are typically high grade and more harmful. *CIS* is always high grade and can be dangerous. *Micropapillary* tumors are always high grade and very dangerous.

The other 10% of bladder cancer cell types, including **squamous cell carcinoma**, **adenocarcinoma**, **small cell carcinoma**, and **sarcoma**, are all high grade and aggressive.

Other Diagnostic Considerations

Other aspects of your diagnosis, such as how many tumors you have, the size of the tumor(s), and the location(s) of the tumor(s), are factors that will be considered by your doctor when determining your treatment options and assessing your prognosis.

What Are My Risks of Recurrence and/or Progression?

Since bladder cancer has a very high rate of recurrence and can progress to a more advanced form of the disease, you need to understand the risks of recurrence and/or progression of your disease.

Recurrence refers to a return of bladder cancer after there is a *complete response* to treatment (no evidence of disease). Both low-grade and high-grade bladder cancer have a high risk of recurrence. The disease can recur in the same or in a different location(s), either as a single tumor or as multiple tumors. There is an increased risk of recurrence if the primary tumor was 3 cm or larger, there were multiple tumors, there was CIS, and/or there was a prior recurrence.

Progression refers to a worsening of bladder cancer to a higher stage and/or grade. The risk of progression is low for patients with low-grade disease. On the other hand, the risk of progression is high for patients with high-grade disease. When bladder cancer invades the muscle, there is a high risk of progression to the lymph nodes and/or distant sites in the body.

YOUR PATHOLOGY REPORT

Diagnosing bladder cancer requires the microscopic examination of a tissue sample (biopsy), which can be a small biopsy or an entire tumor. Based on the examination of this tissue, a pathologist writes a **pathology report**, which your doctor will receive within about 7 to 10 days.

The findings in the pathology report are based on the pathologist's examination of tissue samples (or entire tumor) under a microscope. The pathology report indicates whether the tissue is benign (noncancerous) or malignant (cancerous) and, if cancerous, the grade, stage, and cell type of the disease. In addition, the pathology report indicates how many tumors there are, the size of the tumor(s), and the location(s) of the tumor(s). If the tissue removed is thought to be the entire tumor, the report will indicate whether or not cancer cells are found at the edges (margins) of the tumor to determine if enough of the tumor and surrounding tissue were removed to completely eliminate the cancer.

Your pathology report contains technical medical terminology, since it is a communication between the pathologist and your doctor. You will need your doctor to explain in plain language the meaning of the report. It is important that you ask your doctor any questions about information you do not understand. You should ask for a copy of your pathology report for your records and refer to it when you have questions about your disease.

Based on the information in your pathology report and the results of other tests, such as imaging tests and urine tests, your doctor will recommend treatment options and assess your prognosis.

Should I Get a Second Opinion?

Because getting a complete and accurate diagnosis is so critical, many patients consider seeking the knowledge and advice of more than one doctor. This is called a *second opinion*. Asking for a second opinion to review your initial diagnosis and treatment recommendations is a common and beneficial practice. The more knowledge you have about your diagnosis and treatment options, the more comfortable you will feel about decisions you make about your treatment and care. Some patients are afraid they will offend their current doctor by getting a second opinion. Do not let this fear deter you. Most doctors fully understand the value of a second opinion and are not offended when patients seek one.

In addition to obtaining a second opinion from a urologist or a urologic oncologist, a second opinion could involve a second pathologist to review biopsy slides, a second medical oncologist to recommend chemotherapy options or clinical trials, or a second radiologist to review imaging tests. If you decide you would like to seek a second opinion, you will want to consult doctors who specialize in the diagnosis and treatment of bladder cancer.

If you decide to seek a second opinion, be sure to bring copies of all medical records related to your bladder cancer evaluation and diagnosis, including reports of your diagnostic tests and procedures, including cystoscopies, TURBTs, imaging studies, and urine cytology. Also, when possible, bring copies of CDs of your imaging scans. Under the federal Health Insurance Portability and Accountability Act of 1996 (HIPAA), you have the right to get copies of your medical records from your health care providers. Most health care providers require you to make a written request on forms that you can obtain from their offices.

NEXT STEPS

Once you and your doctor are confident that your diagnosis is accurate and complete, your doctor will explain your treatment options. There are a wide variety of treatments for bladder cancer, which are discussed in the subsequent chapters of this book. Chapter 6 discusses the treatment of *non-muscle-invasive* bladder cancer. Chapter 7 provides an overview of the various treatment options for *muscle-invasive* bladder cancer. Chapters 8, 9, 10, and 11 discuss the treatment of muscle-invasive bladder cancer with a radical cystectomy. Chapter 12 discusses the treatment of muscle-invasive bladder cancer with bladder preservation therapy, an alternative to a radical cystectomy for carefully selected patients with muscle-invasive disease. Chapter 13 discusses the treatment of *metastatic* bladder cancer.

Part 2 consists of **Chapter 6**, which discusses the stages and grades of ***non-muscle-invasive bladder cancer*** — and how they are treated. About 75% of patients have non-muscle-invasive bladder cancer at the time of diagnosis.

CHAPTER 6

Non-Muscle-Invasive Bladder Cancer

Non-muscle-invasive bladder cancer refers to the stages of bladder cancer in which the disease is confined to the bladder lining (urothelium) or has grown through the bladder lining into the lamina propria — but has *not* invaded the muscle layer of the bladder wall. About 75% of patients have non-muscle-invasive bladder cancer at the time of diagnosis. Non-muscle-invasive bladder cancer has a high rate of recurrence — but is usually not life threatening when treated and monitored appropriately.

In the past, doctors have referred to non-muscle-invasive bladder cancer as *superficial*, and you may still hear this term used.

The *stage* and *grade* of non-muscle-invasive bladder cancer are extremely important, because it is these two factors that determine the appropriate treatment for the disease — as well as the risks of recurrence and/or progression.

This chapter answers the following questions about non-muscle-invasive bladder cancer:

- What are the **stages** of non-muscle-invasive bladder cancer?
- What are the **grades** of non-muscle-invasive bladder cancer?
- What are the risks of **recurrence** and/or **progression** of non-muscle-invasive bladder cancer?
- How is non-muscle-invasive bladder cancer **treated**?
- How is non-muscle-invasive bladder cancer **monitored**?

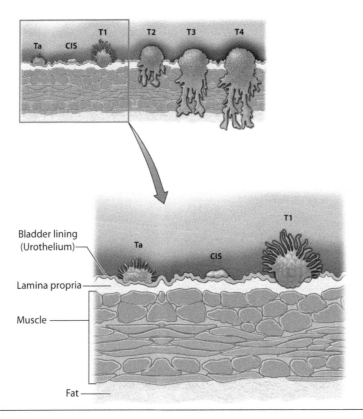

Figure 6.1 Stages of Non-Muscle-Invasive Bladder Cancer

What Are the Stages of Non-Muscle-Invasive Bladder Cancer?

The *stage* of bladder cancer refers to the depth and extent of the tumor. There are three stages of non-muscle-invasive bladder cancer: **Ta**, **CIS** (also called **TIS**), and **T1**. Stages Ta and CIS are confined to the bladder lining (urothelium). Stage T1 has invaded the lamina propria, which is adjacent to the bladder lining (see figure 6.1).

What Are the Grades of Non-Muscle-Invasive Bladder Cancer?

The *grade* of bladder cancer indicates its potential to be aggressive and do harm. Non-muscle-invasive bladder cancer is either low grade or high grade, depending on how the cancer cells appear under a microscope. ***Low-grade*** cancer cells closely resemble normal cells and rarely spread beyond the bladder lining. *High-grade* cancer cells bear little resemblance to normal cells and have a high risk of invading the deeper layers of the bladder wall and spreading to other parts of the body.

What Are the Risks of Recurrence and/or Progression of Non-Muscle-Invasive Bladder Cancer?

Recurrence refers to a return of the cancer after having a *complete response* to treatment (no evidence of disease). Both low-grade bladder cancer and high-grade bladder cancer have a high risk of recurrence.

Progression refers to a worsening of bladder cancer to a higher stage and/or grade. Low-grade bladder cancer has a low risk of progression, whereas high-grade bladder cancer has a high risk of progression.

How Is Non-Muscle-Invasive Bladder Cancer Treated?

There are two main approaches for treating non-muscle-invasive bladder cancer. One involves the surgical resection (removal) of bladder tumors during a **TURBT** or **blue light cystoscopy**. The other approach involves the instillation of drugs into the bladder to kill cancer cells, called **intravesical drug therapy**.

The following discusses the role of TURBT, blue light cystoscopy, and intravesical drug therapy, used individually or in combination, in the treatment of non-muscle-invasive bladder cancer.

TURBT

TURBT stands for **T**rans**U**rethral **R**esection of **B**ladder **T**umor. A TURBT has multiple uses in diagnosing and treating bladder cancer. In chapter 4, we discussed the use of a TURBT (also called **TUR**, which stands for **T**rans**U**rethral **R**esection) for *diagnosing* bladder cancer. In this chapter, we discuss the use of a TURBT for *treating* non-muscle-invasive bladder cancer.

If you have been diagnosed with stage Ta or T1 bladder cancer, the initial treatment is a TURBT to surgically remove all visible cancer. However, a TURBT is not used to treat CIS (carcinoma in situ), a flat tumor, which cannot be removed this way.

A TURBT is performed in an outpatient surgical center or hospital. Once you are in the operating room, you will receive general anesthesia. The doctor uses a *resectoscope* (see chapter 4, figure 4.2), which is passed through your urethra into your bladder. During the TURBT, your doctor is able to see the lining of your bladder under white light. Your doctor views your bladder lining either directly through the lens of the resectoscope or on a television screen.

A resectoscope is equipped with a camera, wide-angle telescope, and channels that permit the passage of small tools into the bladder for the purpose of removing (resecting) bladder tumors. Electricity is the force that removes the tumor (called *electrocauterization* or *fulguration*). A small, electrified, semicircular loop of wire is passed through the resectoscope and moved back and forth through the tumor tissue. Slices of tumor are separated from the lining with each passage of the electrified wire loop, and eventually the entire tumor is disconnected from the bladder lining. The electric loop is also used to cauterize (burn) the tissue and seal blood vessels to stop bleeding from the site where the tumor was removed. After the electric loop is removed, the separated tumor tissue is removed by irrigating the bladder.

A tumor(s) removed during a TURBT is sent to a pathology laboratory to be examined under a microscope by a pathologist. The pathologist writes a pathology report, which is received by your doctor about 7 days after your TURBT. Upon receipt of the report, your doctor will discuss the report with you and determine if further treatment is needed.

The potential side effects and risks of a TURBT are bleeding, pain and/or burning during urination, infection, and bladder perforation. After a TURBT, a catheter (thin, flexible tube) may be placed into the urethra for a day or two to minimize the risk of bleeding, clot formation, and/or over-distention of the bladder.

Blue Light Cystoscopy

A relatively new procedure, called **blue light cystoscopy** (also called *fluorescence cystoscopy*), is increasingly being used to better diagnose patients with suspected or known tumors in the bladder lining. A blue light cystoscopy is similar to a TURBT — but incorporates the instillation of an imaging solution and use of blue light to improve the visualization of tumors. Like a TURBT, a blue light cystoscopy is performed under general anesthesia in an outpatient surgical center or hospital.

In chapter 4, we discussed the use of blue light cystoscopy in diagnosing patients with suspected or known non-muscle-invasive bladder cancer. In this chapter, we discuss how better detection of tumors with blue light cystoscopy can lead to more complete tumor removal and a lower risk of recurrence.

Undergoing a blue light cystoscopy is similar to undergoing a TURBT. However, what makes blue light cystoscopy different from a TURBT is the instillation of an imaging solution, called Cysview®, and the use of blue light in addition to white light for viewing the bladder. About one hour before a blue light cystoscopy, Cysview® is instilled into the bladder through a catheter. The imaging solution contains fluorescent compounds. These compounds absorb fast growing cells, such as cancer cells. When viewed under blue light, the fluorescent compounds that are absorbed by cancer cells appear *red* — allowing better visualization of any cancerous tissue, particularly small or indistinct tumors that may be missed when viewed under white light alone.

The instillation of Cysview® and use of blue light in conjunction with white light can help doctors find more bladder cancer tumors and find them sooner and more completely than with a TURBT using white light alone. Better visualization of tumors can lead to more complete tumor resection (removal), reduced risk of recurrence, and better treatment decisions.

Blue light cystoscopy is well tolerated and considered safe. Side effects and risks associated with blue light cystoscopy are similar to those of a TURBT.

Intravesical Drug Therapy

Another way to treat non-muscle-invasive bladder cancer is with ***intravesical drug therapy*** — that is, with medications instilled into the bladder through a catheter (see figure 6.2).

There are two types of *intravesical* (means *within* or *inside the bladder*) drug therapy: ***intravesical immunotherapy*** and ***intravesical chemotherapy***. Intravesical immunotherapy refers to the instillation of BCG (bacillus Calmette-Guérin) into the bladder. Intravesical chemotherapy refers to the instillation of chemotherapy drugs, such as mitomycin C, into the bladder.

Most intravesical drugs are given on an outpatient basis. A catheter is inserted through the urethra to instill drugs into the bladder. Although the thought of having a catheter inserted through your urethra is not pleasant, most patients tolerate the treatment with minimal discomfort. You will be asked to avoid urinating for up to 2 hours after the drug is instilled into your bladder, so that

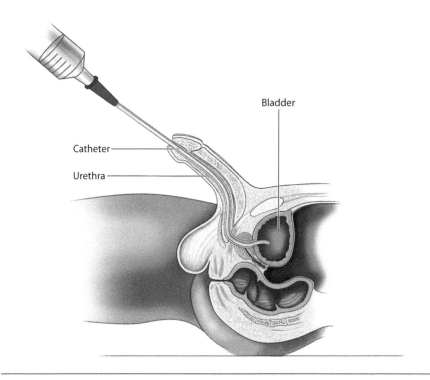

Figure 6.2 Intravesical Drug Therapy

the drug can be held in the bladder and have adequate time to act on the bladder lining. After you empty the drug by urinating, you will be able to resume your normal activities.

BCG (Intravesical Immunotherapy)

BCG is used as a primary treatment for patients with CIS to eradicate the disease and reduce the risks of recurrence and/or progression. BCG is also used as a follow-up treatment after a TURBT for patients with high-grade Ta or T1 disease to eliminate any residual (remaining) disease and reduce the risks of recurrence and/or progression.

BCG works by causing an immune response in the bladder lining. The idea behind any type of immunotherapy is that a person's own immune system can be harnessed for the purpose of killing cancer cells. In patients whose systems are able to mount such a response, the reaction kills cancer cells.

BCG, which was first introduced in the mid-1970s, is made from bacteria related to the organism that causes human tuberculosis. Although BCG is one of the most effective drugs for treating non-muscle-invasive bladder cancer, doctors do not fully understand the mechanism by which it destroys bladder cancer cells.

BCG treatment begins with an *induction* course, which consists of a total of 6 doses of BCG. One dose is administered once a week for 6 weeks. About 4 to 6 weeks after the last dose, the patient undergoes a cystoscopy to assess his or her response to the induction course. Depending on the response, follow-up treatment with BCG may be given. This could consist of a 3-week course of BCG given every 6 months for 3 years. Patients who undergo follow-up BCG treatment have periodic check-ups to monitor for recurrence and/or progression of their disease.

If bladder cancer persists after two successive courses of BCG, it is unlikely that further treatment with BCG will be effective in eradicating the disease. In such cases, doctors may recommend other intravesical drugs (for example, mitomycin C, or BCG plus interferon) — or surgical removal of the bladder (radical cystectomy) to preempt the spread of the cancer to the muscle of the bladder wall and/or other parts of the body.

Patients who receive BCG may experience a variety of side effects, including blood in the urine, an urgent need to urinate, frequent urination, low-grade fever (100°F), and the sensation of coming down with the flu. These side effects can last for up to 12 hours after treatment. Rarely, if a small amount of BCG is absorbed into the bloodstream during instillation of the drug, the patient may experience a high fever (103°F or higher) and signs of a severe infection. This is the most important and potentially dangerous side effect of BCG. Such a reaction would prompt your doctor to treat you with specific antibiotics to combat the BCG medication. Before you receive BCG, your doctor will review the warning signs of such a reaction.

Intravesical Chemotherapy

Mytomycin C and other intravesical chemotherapy drugs may be used to treat non-muscle-invasive bladder cancer when BCG fails to eradicate the disease. Some doctors use intravesical chemotherapy drugs rather than BCG as the initial treatment for non-muscle-invasive disease.

The potential side effects of intravesical chemotherapy drugs include pain in the bladder, painful urination, irritation of the bladder lining, and allergic reactions, such as rashes on the hands, genitals, and other locations. These side effects usually resolve when the therapy is completed.

Ta, CIS, and T1 Tumors: What You Need to Know

The three stages of non-muscle-invasive bladder cancer are Ta, CIS (also called TIS), and T1. The following discusses each stage and how it is treated.

Stage Ta Bladder Cancer

Ta tumors are confined to the bladder lining (urothelium). About 60% of patients with non-muscle-invasive bladder cancer have stage Ta at the time of diagnosis. Ta disease can occur as a single (focal) tumor or as multiple (multifocal) tumors.

What is the grade? Ta tumors can be low grade or high grade. About 70% of Ta tumors are low grade, and about 30% of Ta tumors are high grade.

How are Ta tumors treated? Low-grade Ta tumors are treated by surgically removing (resecting) the tumors during a TURBT or blue light cystoscopy. High-grade Ta tumors are treated by surgically removing tumors during a TURBT or blue light cystoscopy — often followed by BCG to eradicate any residual disease and reduce the risks of recurrence and/or progression.

Ta tumors that occur in combination with CIS are more likely to progress to muscle-invasive disease. Thus, Ta tumors that occur in combination with CIS are treated more aggressively and watched more closely than Ta tumors that occur in the absence of CIS.

What are the risks of recurrence and/or progression? Low-grade Ta tumors have about a 30% chance of recurring and about a 5% chance of progressing. High-grade Ta tumors have about a 70% chance of recurring and about a 20% to 30% chance of progressing.

Although the recurrence of Ta tumors can be a nuisance for patients — requiring additional treatment and the inconvenience that goes with it — it is tumor *progression* that is the major medical threat to people with non-muscle-invasive bladder cancer. Accordingly, doctors tend to treat patients with high-grade Ta tumors more aggressively and follow them more intensively than patients with low-grade Ta tumors.

CIS (Carcinoma in Situ)

CIS is a flat tumor, which may appear as a red velvety patch on the bladder lining. About 10% of patients with non-muscle-invasive bladder cancer have CIS at the time of diagnosis. Unlike a Ta or T1 tumor, CIS is not amenable to surgical resection (removal) during a TURBT or blue light cystoscopy.

CIS can occur by itself or in combination with other tumors, including Ta and T1 tumors. Ta or T1 tumors that occur in combination with CIS are considered more dangerous than Ta or T1 tumors that occur in the absence of CIS.

What is the grade? CIS is always high grade.

How is CIS treated? The most common initial treatment for CIS is BCG, which results in a complete response (no evidence of disease) about 50% to 70% of the time. For patients with CIS who do not have a complete response to BCG, some doctors offer other options for intravesical drug therapy. This can include intravesical chemotherapy drugs, such as mitomycin C, or BCG plus interferon. If CIS persists after intravesical drug therapy, or if CIS recurs after a complete response to intravesical drug therapy, a radical cystectomy is usually recommended to preempt the spread of the disease to the muscle of the bladder wall and/or other parts of the body.

What are the risks of recurrence and/or progression? For patients with CIS who have a complete response to BCG, the risk of recurrence is about 50% and the risk of progression is about 20%. CIS has a reputation for unpredictable behavior — and, in some cases, can spread outside the bladder without apparently invading the muscle.

Stage T1 Bladder Cancer

Some tumors have the ability to penetrate through the bladder lining into the lamina propria. Tumors that invade the lamina propria are called stage T1 tumors. About 30% of patients with non-muscle-invasive bladder cancer have stage T1 at the time of diagnosis.

What is the grade? T1 tumors are almost always high grade. It is not unusual for T1 tumors to occur in combination with CIS, which is a potentially difficult combination to treat.

How are T1 tumors treated? Some experts believe that stage T1 bladder cancer represents not the most invasive form of non-muscle-invasive bladder cancer but rather the least invasive form of muscle-invasive bladder cancer. Having said that, doctors currently categorize tumors that invade the lamina propria (T1 tumors) as non-muscle-invasive. Accordingly, most patients with T1 tumors are treated with standard therapies for non-muscle-invasive bladder cancer — that is, by resecting tumors during a TURBT or blue light cystoscopy, usually followed by BCG to eradicate any residual disease and reduce the risks of recurrence and/or progression. If BCG fails to eradicate T1 disease, some doctors offer other options for intravesical drug therapy. This can include intra-vesical chemotherapy drugs, such as mitomycin C, or BCG plus interferon.

Although many people with T1 disease have a complete response to therapies for non-muscle-invasive bladder cancer, there is a sizeable minority who do not. Those who do not have a complete response to these therapies have as high as a 50% risk of progression to muscle-invasive disease within a year or two of their failure to respond to treatment. This prompts urologists to recommend a radical cystectomy to preempt the spread of the disease to the muscle of the bladder wall and/or other parts of the body.

T1 tumors that occur in combination with CIS are notoriously difficult to control. Some studies suggest that if a patient with a T1 tumor in combination with CIS does not have a complete response after two successive courses of BCG, the likelihood of progression to muscle-invasive bladder cancer is about 50%. Armed with this information, most urologists are reluctant to continue treating these patients with BCG. Instead, most doctors will recommend a radical cystectomy as the safest, most effective way to treat a difficult, treatment-resistant bladder tumor.

What are the risks of recurrence and/or progression? Patients with T1 bladder cancer have about a 70% risk of recurrence and about a 30% risk of progression.

How Is Non-Muscle-Invasive Bladder Cancer Monitored?

Once your cancer has been treated, your urologist will need to keep a watchful eye on your bladder. No matter which type of treatment you receive, one thing is certain: You will need to be monitored closely for many years, probably the rest of your life, to make sure that if your cancer comes back — as bladder cancer often does — it will be detected and treated as early as possible. This surveillance usually includes a cystoscopy or blue light cystoscopy at sched-uled intervals. In the United States, the standard schedule for surveillance is a cystoscopy every 3 months for 2 years following diagnosis and, subsequently, every 6 months for an additional 2 years. If after 4 years of surveillance no tumors are detected, the intervals between follow-up visits may be increased to follow-up visits once a year. The goal of surveillance is to detect and treat tumor recurrences early, when the cancer is most amenable to treatment and less likely to do harm.

PART 3 TREATMENTS FOR MUSCLE-INVASIVE BLADDER CANCER

Part 3 consists of **Chapters 7–12**, which discuss *muscle-invasive bladder cancer* and its treatment. About 20% of patients have muscle-invasive bladder cancer at the time of diagnosis.

Chapter 7 is an introduction to muscle-invasive bladder cancer. **Chapters 8–11** discuss the standard treatment for muscle-invasive bladder cancer, called a *radical cystectomy*. **Chapter 12** discusses *bladder preservation therapy*, a treatment approach for selected patients with muscle-invasive bladder cancer. Another name for bladder preservation therapy is *bladder-sparing therapy* or *trimodality therapy (TMT)*.

CHAPTER 7

Introduction to Muscle-Invasive Bladder Cancer

Once bladder cancer has invaded the muscle layer of the bladder wall, it is called *muscle-invasive* bladder cancer. Muscle-invasive bladder cancer also refers to disease that has invaded the fat around the muscle and/or has extended to nearby organs, such as the prostrate in men or the vagina or uterus in women. About 20% of bladder cancer patients have muscle-invasive bladder cancer at the time of diagnosis.

This chapter discusses the stages and grade of muscle-invasive bladder cancer and introduces the different treatment options for muscle-invasive bladder cancer (discussed in detail in chapters 8–12).

What Are the Stages of Muscle-Invasive Bladder Cancer?

The *stage* of bladder cancer refers to the depth and extent of the tumor. The stages of muscle-invasive bladder cancer are **T2**, **T3**, and **T4a** (see figure 7.1). A tumor that has invaded the muscle of the bladder wall is stage T2. A tumor that has penetrated through the muscle of the bladder wall to the fat surrounding the muscle is stage T3. A tumor that has extended to organs adjacent to the bladder, such as the prostate in men or the vagina or uterus in women, is stage T4a — also referred to as *locally advanced disease*. Although stages T3 and T4a extend beyond the muscle, they are included in the muscle-invasive category because they are treated the same as muscle-invasive disease.

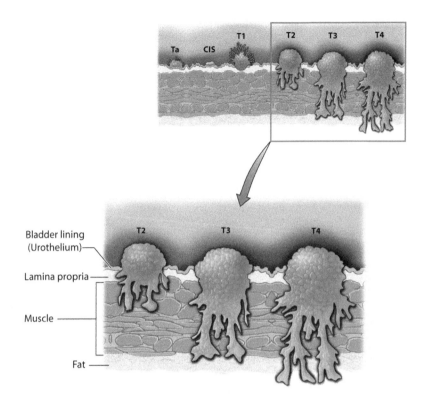

Figure 7.1 Stages of Muscle-Invasive Bladder Cancer

Stage **T4b** bladder cancer has invaded the rectum, abdominal wall, or pelvic wall. This stage of bladder cancer — like metastatic bladder cancer — is treated with systemic drugs. Given that T4b is treated like metastatic bladder cancer (systemic disease), T4b is categorized as metastatic bladder cancer.

What Is the Grade of Muscle-Invasive Bladder Cancer?

The *grade* of bladder cancer indicates its potential to be aggressive and do harm. All stages of muscle-invasive bladder cancer are ***high grade***, which is a high-risk, aggressive form of the disease. Muscle-invasive bladder cancer has the potential to metastasize to lymph nodes and distant sites, because the muscle layer of the bladder wall contains lymphatic vessels that act as interconnecting highways for the spread of the disease to other parts of the body.

What Are the Treatment Options for Muscle-Invasive Bladder Cancer?

The following are the different treatment options for muscle-invasive bladder cancer. These treatment options are discussed in detail in chapters 8–12.

Radical Cystectomy: A radical cystectomy is the "gold standard" treatment for muscle-invasive bladder cancer. A radical cystectomy is the surgical removal of the bladder and reconstruction of the lower urinary tract to provide a way for urine to be eliminated after the bladder is removed. Chapters 8, 9, 10, and 11 discuss a radical cystectomy — including the decision to have a radical cystectomy, what is involved in undergoing the surgery, choosing a urinary tract reconstruction, and recovery after a radical cystectomy.

Partial Cystectomy: A partial cystectomy is a treatment option for about 5% of patients with muscle-invasive bladder cancer. A partial cystectomy removes only a portion of the bladder, leaving the remainder of the bladder intact. Chapter 8 includes a discussion of a partial cystectomy.

Bladder Preservation Therapy: Bladder preservation therapy is a treatment option for carefully selected patients with muscle-invasive bladder cancer. Bladder preservation therapy, also called *bladder-sparing therapy* or *trimodality therapy (TMT)*, treats the cancer without removing the bladder. The therapy begins with a TURBT, followed by systemic chemotherapy and radiation given concurrently, called *chemoradiation*. Chapter 12 discusses bladder preservation therapy.

CHAPTER 8

The Decision to Have a Radical Cystectomy

The "gold standard" treatment for patients with muscle-invasive bladder cancer is a *radical cystectomy*. This surgical procedure involves removal of the bladder and reconstruction of the lower urinary tract to provide a way for urine to be collected and eliminated after the bladder is removed.

If you are considering a radical cystectomy, you are likely to have questions about the surgery and what it means for your survival and quality of life. This is the first of four chapters (8, 9, 10, and 11) that discusses a radical cystectomy. Topics include the decision to have the surgery (this chapter), what is involved in undergoing a radical cystectomy (chapter 9), what you need to know to choose a urinary tract reconstruction (chapter 10), and recovery after a radical cystectomy (chapter 11).

This chapter answers the following questions patients have when considering a radical cystectomy:

- When is a radical cystectomy indicated?
- Who is a candidate for a radical cystectomy?
- What is involved in the decision to have a radical cystectomy?
- What are the benefits of a radical cystectomy?
- What are the risks of a radical cystectomy?
- What are the other treatment options?

When Is a Radical Cystectomy Indicated?

A radical cystectomy is the standard treatment for bladder cancer that has invaded the muscle layer of the bladder wall. Once the cancer has invaded the muscle, there is a high risk the cancer will spread (metastasize) outside the bladder to surrounding lymph nodes, nearby organs and structures, and/or distant parts of the body, such as the liver, lung, or bone. Once the disease has spread beyond the bladder, treatment and cure become much more difficult.

A radical cystectomy is usually not offered to patients whose cancer has spread to the lymph nodes and/or distant sites, such as the liver, lung, or bone. Bladder cancer that has spread to these areas, called *metastatic* bladder cancer, is treated with systemic chemotherapy (cancer drugs delivered intravenously).

Although a radical cystectomy is the standard treatment for muscle-invasive bladder cancer (stages T2–T4a), it may also be appropriate for stages T1 and CIS (carcinoma in situ) that do not respond to standard therapies for non-muscle-invasive disease (discussed in chapter 6).

Who Is a Candidate for a Radical Cystectomy?

The criteria for patient selection for a radical cystectomy include the stage of the cancer, the patient's age and overall health, and if there is a co-existing medical condition(s) that increases the risk associated with the surgery. To determine if you are a candidate for a radical cystectomy, your doctor will perform a thorough evaluation, including a review of your medical history, a physical examination, a TURBT, and imaging tests. The following discusses the role of a TURBT and imaging tests in this evaluation.

TURBT

Your doctor will perform a TURBT to assess whether your cancer invades the muscle layer of the bladder wall, which is the most common indication that you need a radical cystectomy. Most likely you had a TURBT at the time of your initial diagnosis, so why is your doctor recommending that you have another TURBT? Several months may have passed since your last TURBT, and your doctor needs to reassess the stage of your disease. Furthermore, your initial

TURBT may not have included a sample of muscle tissue, or there may not have been enough muscle tissue in the sample to make an accurate assessment of whether you have muscle-invasive disease.

An additional TURBT, sometimes referred to as a *restaging* TURBT, can turn up new information, such as the discovery of residual cancer that was not found at the time of the initial TURBT. Studies show that in nearly 60% of people diagnosed with muscle-invasive bladder cancer, a restaging TURBT provides additional information that indicates either an increase in the stage (the cancer is more extensive than previously thought), or a decrease in the stage (the cancer is less extensive than previously thought). In either case, a restaging TURBT provides the most current information upon which to base a treatment recommendation.

Imaging Tests

Your evaluation for a radical cystectomy will often include imaging tests, such as a CT scan or an MRI scan, to assess whether cancer has spread outside your bladder. As mentioned above, a radical cystectomy is usually not offered to patients whose cancer has metastasized (spread) to the lymph nodes and/or distant parts of the body.

What Is Involved in the Decision to Have a Radical Cystectomy?

Once you learn that you are a suitable candidate for a radical cystectomy, you will no doubt have many questions to discuss with your doctor, including the potential benefits and risks associated with the surgery. You will want to compare the benefits and risks of a radical cystectomy with those of other possible treatment options. For selected patients with muscle-invasive bladder cancer, other treatment options may include a partial cystectomy (discussed later in this chapter) or bladder preservation therapy (mentioned briefly later in this chapter and discussed in detail in chapter 12).

You may want to get a second opinion to help you gather as much information as possible before making a treatment decision. Ultimately, the therapy you choose is a personal decision based on your specific diagnosis and your treatment goals and preferences.

What Are the Benefits of a Radical Cystectomy?

The potential benefits of a radical cystectomy are long-term survival and cure. Patients whose disease is confined to the bladder (stages T1 and T2) have the best long-term survival rates after a radical cystectomy (see figure 8.1).

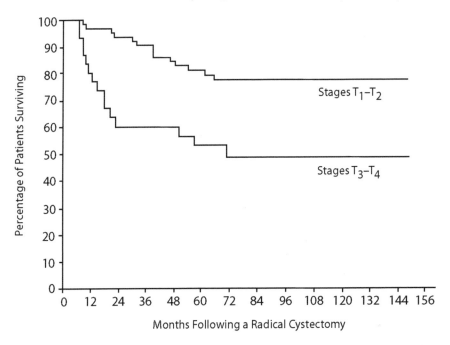

Survival Rates By Stage After a Radical Cystectomy

Bladder cancer (disease-specific) survival rates by stage for patients after undergoing a radical cystectomy at Johns Hopkins. Patients were followed for at least 10 years. Reprinted from Schoenberg et al., "Local Recurrence and Survival Following Nerve Sparing Radical Cystoprostatectomy for Bladder Cancer: 10-Year Followup," *Journal of Urology* 1996, 155(2): 490–494.

Figure 8.1 Survival Rates by Stage After a Radical Cystectomy

What Are the Risks of a Radical Cystectomy?

As with any major surgery, there are risks associated with a radical cystectomy. Up to 70% of patients who undergo this surgery will experience one or more side effects or complications related to the procedure. Many of the risks are the same as those associated with any major surgery, such as the need for a blood transfusion, bleeding, blood clot(s), pulmonary embolism, bowel obstruction, infection, fever, injury to other organs, failure to cure, or death due to complications of the surgery. Other risks, such as sexual dysfunction, infertility, and incontinence, are also related to a radical cystectomy (see chapters 10 and 11).

What Are the Other Treatment Options?

It is important that you consider all of your treatment options before making a decision. Other treatment options for selected patients with muscle-invasive disease are a *partial cystectomy* and *bladder preservation therapy*.

Partial Cystectomy

About 5% of patients with muscle-invasive bladder cancer are candidates for a **partial cystectomy**, a surgical procedure in which only a portion of the bladder is removed. With this option, bladder function is preserved.

The criteria for selecting patients for a partial cystectomy include the following:

- It is the patient's first bladder tumor.
- The tumor is small, and there is only one tumor.
- There is no CIS (carcinoma in situ).
- The tumor is in a location in the bladder, such as the dome, such that the portion of the bladder that will be removed will not interfere with the bladder's ability to function.
- The remainder of the bladder is completely free of cancer cells.

Because the vast majority of patients with muscle-invasive bladder cancer do not meet these criteria, it is unlikely that you will be offered a partial cystectomy if you have muscle-invasive disease. However, for patients who are suitable candidates for this treatment, a partial cystectomy can result in excellent long-term survival and disease control.

Bladder Preservation Therapy

Another treatment option for selected patients with muscle-invasive bladder cancer is **bladder preservation therapy,** also called **bladder-sparing therapy** or **trimodality therapy (TMT).** This approach treats the cancer without removing the bladder. It begins with a TURBT, followed by systemic chemotherapy and radiation therapy given concurrently, called *chemoradiation.*

Careful patient selection is key to achieving good outcomes with this approach. You will need to consult with a urologic oncologist, preferably at a cancer center that treats a high volume of patients with bladder preservation therapy, to determine if you are a suitable candidate for this treatment approach. (See chapter 12 for a detailed discussion of bladder preservation therapy.)

CHAPTER 9

Undergoing a Radical Cystectomy

After careful consideration of your treatment options, you may decide that a radical cystectomy offers you the best chance of achieving a cure, despite the risks associated with the surgery. In anticipation of a radical cystectomy, you will have many questions about how to prepare for the surgery, what is involved in undergoing the operation, and what you will learn about your disease from your postoperative pathology report.

Preparing for a Radical Cystectomy

Your surgeon and other members of your medical team will play a key role in helping you prepare for your surgery. Questions to ask and topics to discuss with your surgeon prior to surgery include the following:

- What are my options for urinary tract reconstruction — and how should I go about choosing an option?
- Will neoadjuvant chemotherapy be recommended prior to the surgery?
- What preoperative tests and examinations will I need?
- Should I donate my own blood before the surgery in the event I need a blood transfusion?
- What is the protocol for bowel preparation before the surgery?
- When will I meet with an enterostomal therapy (ET) nurse?
- When will I meet with an anesthesiologist?

What Are My Options for Urinary Tract Reconstruction — and How Should I Go About Choosing an Option?

A radical cystectomy involves surgical removal of the bladder and reconstruction of the lower urinary tract, called **urinary tract reconstruction**. Reconstruction of the lower urinary tract is necessary after bladder removal to provide a way for urine to be collected and eliminated after the bladder is removed.

There are three types of urinary tract reconstructions: an **ileal conduit**, an **orthotopic neobladder** (also called **neobladder**), and a **continent catheterizable reservoir**. These reconstructions are also referred to as *urinary diversions*. You will need to consult with your surgeon and other members of your medical team about the type of urinary tract reconstruction you want performed during your radical cystectomy.

Choosing from among your options for urinary tract reconstruction is one of the most important decisions you will have to make before your surgery. To make an informed decision, you will need to understand each of your options and how it will affect your life. See chapter 10 for a detailed discussion of what you need to know to choose a urinary tract reconstruction, including how the different types of reconstructions work, how they are constructed, the risks and complications associated with each type of reconstruction, and things to consider when comparing urinary tract reconstructions.

Will Neoadjuvant Chemotherapy Be Recommended Prior to the Surgery?

For patients diagnosed with muscle-invasive bladder cancer, there is about a 20% to 30% chance that cancer cells have spread outside the bladder to surrounding lymph nodes and/or distant sites, but the tumors are too small to be detected by imaging tests. These hidden (occult) tumors are called *micrometastases*, also called *micrometastatic* disease. The higher the tumor stage, the higher the risk of micrometastatic disease.

The use of systemic chemotherapy (drugs given intravenously to attack cancer cells throughout the body) prior to a radical cystectomy is called **neoadjuvant** *chemotherapy*. There is evidence that this approach improves survival after a radical cystectomy. However, there continue to be varying opinions among doctors about the relative risks and benefits of giving neoadjuvant chemotherapy before a radical cystectomy. You will need to discuss this option with your doctor.

What Preoperative Tests and Examinations Will I Need?

The preparation for a radical cystectomy is similar to the preparation required before any major surgery. Most patients are required to visit their primary care doctor for a complete preoperative physical examination, which includes routine blood tests, an electrocardiogram (EKG) of the heart, and a chest X-ray. If you have any co-existing medical condition(s), such as heart disease, you may have to consult with other specialist(s) to evaluate your risks related to the surgery. Based on your preoperative evaluation, your surgeon will tell you if you are approved for the surgery and if there are any limitations on your options for urinary tract reconstruction.

Should I Donate My Own Blood Before the Surgery in the Event I Need a Blood Transfusion?

As many as 30% of patients require a blood transfusion to replace the blood lost during a radical cystectomy. Some patients elect to donate their own blood prior to the surgery to avoid the need for a transfusion of blood obtained from someone else. In an era of heightened awareness about transfusion-related disease, such as HIV and hepatitis C, this approach seems sensible, but it can be inconvenient and sometimes debilitating for older patients. The risk of contracting HIV from a blood transfusion is now considered to be 1 in 1.8 million, and the risk of contracting hepatitis C is about 1 in 100,000. Since the blood supply is relatively safe, most people do not choose to donate their own blood prior to a radical cystectomy, although some will insist upon doing so for their own peace of mind. There is no right answer to the question of whether or not you should donate your own blood. This is a personal matter that you should discuss with your surgeon.

When Will I Meet with an Enterostomal Therapy (ET) Nurse?

Regardless of the type of urinary tract reconstruction you choose, you will need to meet with an ET nurse before your surgery to choose a location for a *stoma,* a surgical opening created in the abdominal wall through which urine can exit the body. An ET nurse, also called an *enterostomal therapist* or *ostomy nurse,* is trained to care for people with stomas.

The two types of urinary tract reconstructions that require a stoma are an ileal conduit and a continent catheterizable reservoir. The only type of urinary tract reconstruction that does not require a stoma is a neobladder. However, even if you choose a neobladder, you will still have to choose a location for a stoma prior to your surgery. This is because your surgeon may learn during your surgery that you are not a suitable candidate for a neobladder. In this case, your doctor would need to create either an ileal conduit or a continent catheterizable reservoir — which both require a stoma.

To assist you in choosing the location for your stoma, the ET nurse will examine your abdomen for scars, skin folds, and location of belt line, and observe what changes occur in your contours as you sit, stand, and bend. It is important that you be able to see and reach your stoma easily. A well-placed and well-constructed stoma will reduce the risk of postoperative complications and speed the recovery process.

What Is the Protocol for Bowel Preparation Before the Surgery?

In preparation for a radical cystectomy, the traditional approach has been to get the bowel as clean as possible, with the idea that anything less could raise the risk of infection when tissue from the intestine(s) is used during urinary tract reconstruction. However, at some hospitals, this practice is changing. Many surgeons favor less extensive bowel preparation, and some surgeons believe that no bowel preparation is better.

When Will I Meet with an Anesthesiologist?

In preparation for a radical cystectomy, you will meet with an anesthesiologist, a doctor who specializes in giving drugs or other agents to prevent pain during surgery. It is the job of the anesthesiologist to inform you about different options for complete pain control during your surgery. Most patients who undergo a radical cystectomy are given general anesthesia. Some patients, for health reasons, may require spinal anesthesia instead, although this is unusual.

General anesthesia refers to the use of anesthetic drugs, which are used to keep patients from feeling any pain during surgery. A general anesthetic also causes a complete loss of awareness during surgery, which patients experience as a kind of deep sleep. *Spinal anesthesia* refers to anesthetic drugs injected into the fluid in the lower part of the spinal column, which causes a temporary loss of feeling in the abdomen during surgery. Patients who receive spinal anesthesia are awake during surgery.

On the day of your surgery, before you go into the operating room, you will have a final meeting with the anesthesiologist to discuss the type of anesthesia that will be used during the procedure.

What Is Involved in Undergoing a Radical Cystectomy?

Operating rooms vary in appearance from hospital to hospital. However, all operating rooms share certain common characteristics. Bright lights illuminate the room to help surgeons see inside the body. The temperature in operating rooms tends to be kept cool, because the surgical team wears heavy gowns and multiple layers of clothing to ensure sterility during surgery. To keep the patient warm during surgery, specially designed heating blankets are applied to the parts of the patient's body not involved in the operation.

The operating room is full of equipment, including monitors that the anesthesiologist uses to ensure that the patient is safely asleep throughout the operation. Nurses and surgical assistants set up equipment and instruments and arrange all of the tools necessary for performing the operation. Everyone wears special scrub suits, caps, and masks to help keep the equipment from being contaminated.

You will be asked to lie down on an operating table and will be covered with warm blankets. The anesthesiologist will administer a sedative to relax you and enable you to drift off to sleep. You will have an endotracheal tube (a breathing tube) placed in your mouth after you are under light anesthesia to ensure that you get enough oxygen during the operation. You will probably not recall having this tube, as it will most likely be removed as soon as you start to wake up from the operation. The only sign of it may be a lingering sore throat for a few days.

Once you are asleep, your body will be prepared for surgery. Your gown will be removed, and your abdomen and genital area will be shaved. Specialized soap designed to kill bacteria will be applied to the skin of your abdomen to minimize the risk of infection after the surgery. Sterile sheets will be placed all around you, and the operation will begin.

The Surgical Procedure

Most surgeons perform a radical cystectomy through an incision that runs from just below the umbilicus (belly button) to the bone above the genitalia. The incision is made down through the layers of the abdominal wall to reveal the internal cavity in which many of the abdominal organs are located.

The surgeon then removes lymph nodes from the vicinity of the bladder and sends them to the pathology laboratory to be tested for cancer cells. This can be done in about 20 minutes. If the pathologist tells the surgeon that cancer cells are present in the lymph node(s), the surgeon may elect to stop the operation. However, on this point there is disagreement among surgeons. Many doctors will proceed with the surgery even if cancer is detected in one or more lymph node(s). Prior to the surgery, it is important to discuss with your doctor under what circumstances he or she would stop the operation. If your doctor elects to stop the operation, he or she will likely recommend systemic chemotherapy before reconsidering bladder removal surgery.

After removal of the lymph nodes, the bladder is removed. In all male patients, the prostate is also removed. In some female patients, a portion of the vagina, the uterus, the cervix, the fallopian tubes, and/or the ovaries may be removed.

The last phase of the surgery is the reconstruction of the lower urinary tract, called *urinary tract reconstruction*, to provide a way for urine to leave the body after the bladder is removed. Your doctor will create a urinary tract reconstruction — either an ileal conduit, a neobladder, or a continent catheterizable reservoir (see chapter 10 for a detailed discussion of the options for urinary tract reconstruction).

When you awaken from the operation, you will have one or two drains coming out of your abdomen next to the incision made during surgery. These drains are usually connected to vacuum reservoirs and serve to evacuate blood clots and remove excess fluid that accumulates in the vicinity of the incision. These drains will remain in place during your hospital stay.

If you have an ileal conduit, an external pouch, called an *ostomy bag*, will be attached with an adhesive to the skin around your stoma before you leave the operating room. The ostomy bag collects urine as it drains from the stoma.

If you have a neobladder, a catheter (tube), often called a *Foley* catheter, will be inserted through your urethra into your neobladder before you leave the operating room. Urine will drain through the catheter while your neobladder is healing.

If you have a continent catheterizable reservoir, two catheters (tubes) will be inserted into your continent catheterizable reservoir before you leave the operating room. One of the catheters, called a *stoma* catheter, will be inserted through your newly created stoma. The other catheter, called a *suprapubic* catheter, will be inserted through your abdominal wall. Urine will drain through the catheters while your continent catheterizable reservoir is healing.

Other Information About a Radical Cystectomy

The removal of the bladder and reconstruction of the lower urinary tract usually takes 3 to 5 hours. Keep in mind, however, that the preparation prior to the beginning of surgery usually takes about 30 minutes and additional time is required after the surgery to apply a sterile bandage to your incision site, awaken you from anesthesia, and then transport you to the recovery room. Thus, the entire process from beginning to end could take anywhere from 4 to 7 hours.

THE *da Vinci*® SURGICAL SYSTEM FOR A RADICAL CYSTECTOMY

In the past decade, the landscape of American surgery has been transformed by the introduction of the *da Vinci*® Surgical System. This is a minimally invasive robotic procedure that a surgeon performs by inserting instruments through small incisions (openings) in the body's abdominal wall. The system's robotic arms permit the surgeon to control the position and function of specially designed tools for pelvic surgery. The *da Vinci*® Surgical System is now commonly used to perform surgery to remove the prostate (a radical prostatectomy) for patients with prostate cancer. In recent years, an increasing number of surgeons are using the *da Vinci*® Surgical System to perform all or part of a radical cystectomy.

The use of the *da Vinci*® Surgical System to perform a radical cystectomy is considered by some to be experimental and by others to be just another way of performing the surgery. No matter which camp your urologist is in, several facts are accepted about the *da Vinci*® Surgical System. It is considered safe in the hands of an experienced surgeon and is associated with a lower amount of blood loss compared to a traditional open radical cystectomy. Surgery performed with the *da Vinci*® takes longer than open operations and costs the health care system more because of the increased operating time and cost of the equipment. The complication rates appear to be the same for a radical cystectomy performed with the *da Vinci*® Surgical System as for a traditional open radical cystectomy.

As is often the case with surgery, the quality of the surgery and the surgeon are more important than which tools he or she chooses to accomplish the job. You should be mindful of suggestions that a robotic surgical system is in any way superior to open surgery, except with respect to blood loss. There are no data to support the claim that outcomes with robotic surgery are better than those achieved with conventional open surgery. If your surgeon suggests using the *da Vinci*® Surgical System, find out about your doctor's personal experience with this new technology, how many surgeries he or she has performed using it, and what the outcomes have been.

After you arrive in the recovery room, further time will be required to ensure that your condition is stable.

For family members waiting in the visitors' room for a loved one undergoing surgery, the wait can be a long one. In many hospitals, nurses and operating room staff attempt to keep family members updated by phoning the waiting room or visiting with the patient's family during the surgery. You should ask your surgeon about such practices at the hospital where you plan to have the surgery. Communication during the procedure can be reassuring to all involved.

Your Postoperative Pathology Report

The organs and tissues removed during your radical cystectomy are sent to a pathology laboratory to be examined by a pathologist. Your surgeon will receive your pathology report within about 7 to 10 days after the surgery. If your pathology report indicates that cancer cells were found outside the bladder in surrounding lymph node(s) or nearby organs or structures, you will most likely be offered systemic chemotherapy after the surgery, called *adjuvant chemotherapy*. If your doctor recommends this therapy, he or she will refer you to a medical oncologist, a doctor who specializes in treating bladder cancer with systemic chemotherapy.

CHAPTER 10

Choosing a Urinary Tract Reconstruction

Your surgeon will create a ***urinary tract reconstruction*** during your radical cystectomy to provide a way for urine to be collected and eliminated after your bladder is removed. There are three types of urinary tract reconstructions: an ***ileal conduit***, an ***orthotopic neobladder***, and a ***continent catheterizable reservoir***. Another name for urinary tract reconstruction is *urinary diversion*.

Choosing a urinary tract reconstruction is one of the most important decisions you will have to make prior to your surgery. Your surgeon and other members of your medical team will play a key role in educating you about your options for urinary tract reconstruction. In addition, it may be helpful to talk with patients with the type of urinary tract reconstruction(s) you are considering to gain additional information from a patient's perspective.

Factors that determine your options for urinary tract reconstruction include your age and general health, the extent of your disease, and any co-existing medical conditions, such as bowel or kidney disease, that may rule out a particular type of reconstruction. Your surgeon will determine if you are a candidate for all three types of urinary tract reconstructions or whether your options for reconstruction are limited.

When choosing a urinary tract reconstruction, it is important to carefully consider your reconstruction options — and the potential impact of each type of reconstruction on your life.

This chapter answers the following questions about the three types of urinary tract reconstructions:

- How do they work?
- How are they constructed?
- What are the risks and complications associated with each type of urinary tract reconstruction?
- What are things to consider about each type of urinary tract reconstruction when deciding which one is best for you?

Ileal Conduit

An **ileal conduit** is the oldest and most commonly used urinary tract reconstruction in the United States today (see figure 10.1). It is called an *incontinent* urinary tract reconstruction because it does not store urine inside the body.

In discussions about an ileal conduit, you will hear the terms *ostomy, stoma,* and *ostomy bag.* An ostomy is a procedure that creates a surgical opening (hole) from the inside to the outside of the body. This opening is called a *stoma* or an *ostomy.* Urine exits the body through the stoma. The urine collects in an external pouch, called an *ostomy bag,* which is attached with an adhesive to the skin around the stoma.

How Does an Ileal Conduit Work?

Urine is produced in the kidneys and passes through the ureters — just as before the operation. From the ureters, urine flows into a newly created channel, called an *ileal conduit.* The ileal conduit is attached at one end to the ureters and at the other end to a stoma in the abdomen. Urine travels from the ureters through the ileal conduit and exits the body through the stoma.

An ostomy bag is placed over the stoma to collect urine as it drains through the stoma. The ostomy bag is attached to the skin around the stoma with a special adhesive to prevent urine from leaking onto the skin. The bag must be emptied every 4 to 6 hours and replaced every 2 to 4 days.

An *enterostomal therapy (ET) nurse,* also called an *ostomy nurse,* is trained to care for patients with stomas. If you have an ileal conduit, your ET nurse will teach you how to care for your stoma and change and empty your ostomy bag (discussed in chapter 11).

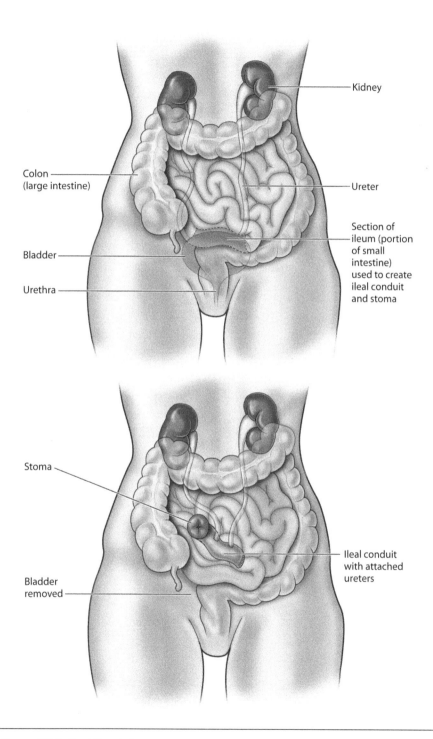

Kidney

Colon
(large intestine)

Ureter

Section of
ileum (portion
of small
intestine)
used to create
ileal conduit
and stoma

Bladder

Urethra

Stoma

Ileal conduit
with attached
ureters

Bladder
removed

Figure 10.1 Ileal Conduit

How Is an Ileal Conduit Constructed?

The surgeon uses a section of the ileum (a portion of the small intestine) to form a channel, called an *ileal conduit*. One end of the ileal conduit is attached to the ureters. The surgeon then creates a small opening, called a *stoma*, in the abdominal wall (usually on the right side). The other end of the ileal conduit is brought through the opening, turned back over the skin around the opening, and stitched to the skin. This provides a way for urine to flow from the ureters into the ileal conduit and exit the body through the stoma. After construction of the ileal conduit and stoma, the surgeon reattaches the remaining intestinal tract to permit normal digestion and bowel movements.

What Are the Risks and Complications Associated with an Ileal Conduit?

Long-term complications related to an ileal conduit include chronic urinary tract infection; slow but steady deterioration of kidney function due to kidney stone formation; a condition called *reflux*, whereby urine washes back into the kidneys, disturbing normal kidney function; scar formation where the ureters are attached to the ileal conduit, leading to obstruction of urine flow into the ileal conduit and subsequent kidney damage; scar formation where the stoma is created in the abdominal wall, leading to obstruction of urine flow out of the ileal conduit and subsequent kidney damage; hernia development adjacent to the stoma; and intermittent bowel obstruction.

Although there is a long list of potential problems associated with an ileal conduit, most patients do well with this type of reconstruction.

Things to Consider About an Ileal Conduit

- An ileal conduit requires a stoma.
- An ileal conduit is the only type of reconstruction that requires an ostomy bag.
- Because urine is not stored inside the body with this type of reconstruction, incontinence is not an issue with an ileal conduit.
- An ileal conduit is the simplest type of reconstruction, involving less operating time, fewer complications during and after surgery, and

shorter recovery time. If you have co-existing medical conditions that raise the risks of undergoing a more complex type of urinary tract reconstruction, you may be better served with an ileal conduit.

• For more information about living with an ileal conduit, see "For Patients with an Ileal Conduit: Caring for Your Stoma" in chapter 11.

Orthotopic Neobladder

An *orthotopic neobladder* (hereafter called **neobladder**) is the urinary tract reconstruction that most closely approximates the body's normal urinary system (see figure 10.2). *Orthotopic* means *in the same place* and *neobladder* means *new bladder*. Essentially, a neobladder is a new bladder created to replace and function like the original bladder. It is called a *continent* urinary tract reconstruction because it stores urine inside the body.

How Does a Neobladder Work?

Urine is produced in the kidneys and passes through the ureters — just as before the operation. From the ureters, urine flows into a newly created internal reservoir, called a *neobladder*, which has the capacity to store urine for about 4 to 6 hours. When you urinate, the urine passes from your neobladder through your urethra to the outside of your body.

A neobladder is not the same as a native bladder. Unlike a native bladder, a neobladder lacks a muscular wall and nerve connections to the brain that facilitate urination. Learning to urinate with a neobladder is often a gradual process, requiring the use of the abdominal and pelvic muscles. As your body recovers from surgery and gets accustomed to your neobladder, you may experience temporary incontinence (lack of urinary control) and need to wear an undergarment pad for a period of time. In most patients, the incontinence will gradually diminish, but this can be a slow process that can take as long as a year or two to completely resolve.

Most people with a neobladder first regain urinary control in the daytime, whereas nighttime continence generally takes longer to regain. In the beginning, you will need to empty your neobladder about every 2 hours, including at night; and you may need to set an alarm clock to comply with this schedule.

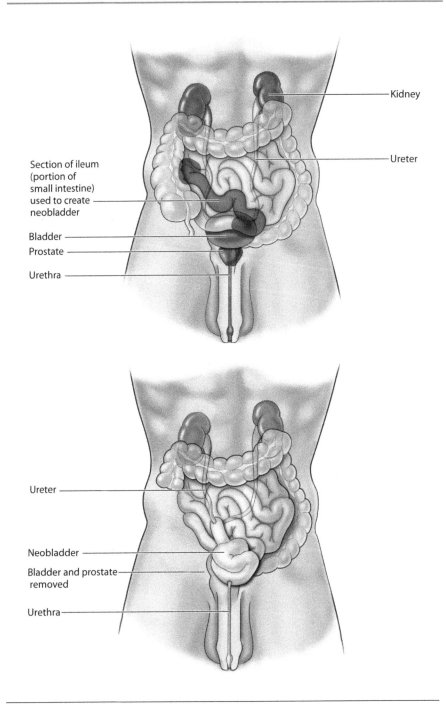

Figure 10.2 Orthotopic Neobladder

As your neobladder heals and increases in size, you will be able to wait longer between emptying — about every 4 to 6 hours.

How Is a Neobladder Constructed?

To construct a neobladder, the surgeon uses a section of the ileum (a portion of the small intestine) to form an internal reservoir. The surgeon attaches the neobladder to the ureters and to the urethra. After constructing a neobladder, the surgeon reattaches the remaining intestinal tract to permit normal digestion and bowel movements.

To construct a neobladder, the surgeon must attach the patient's urethra to the neobladder, so it is imperative that the urethra be free of cancer cells. Therefore, before constructing a neobladder, the surgeon must obtain biopsies from the urethra and send them to the pathology laboratory for examination under a microscope to determine if cancer is present. In order to safely construct a neobladder, the surgeon must remove all cancer from the urethra and still retain enough of the urethra to attach to the neobladder. Otherwise, the patient is disqualified from having a neobladder, and must have another type of reconstruction — either an ileal conduit or a continent catheterizable reservoir. The patient could also be disqualified from having a neobladder because of anatomic reasons. If a neobladder is your first choice of reconstruction, you will need to discuss these possibilities with your doctor before your surgery, so you and your doctor can agree on the type of reconstruction you will have if you cannot have a neobladder.

What Are the Risks and Complications Associated with a Neobladder?

A neobladder is associated with potential risks and complications, the most common of which is *incontinence* — the inability to control urine flow. Incontinence occurs in about 15% of male neobladder patients of any age, about 10% to 15% of female neobladder patients under age 70, and about 30% to 40% of female neobladder patients over age 70. For both men and women, treatment options for incontinence include behavioral changes, Kegel exercises, and an artificial urinary sphincter (AUS), which can be surgically implanted to restore continence.

Another complication associated with a neobladder is *urinary retention*, which is the inability to adequately empty urine from the neobladder when urinating. Urinary retention occurs in about 5% of male neobladder patients and as many as 30% to 40% of female neobladder patients. Patients with urinary retention must insert a catheter through their urethra to empty urine from their neobladder. This is called *self-catheterization*.

Other potential complications associated with a neobladder include scar formation at the attachment of the ureters or urethra to the neobladder, resulting in the obstruction of urine flow; kidney stone formation; chronic urinary tract infection; and intermittent bowel obstruction.

Things to Consider About a Neobladder

- A neobladder allows you to urinate through your urethra without the need for an ostomy bag.
- Learning to urinate with a neobladder is usually a gradual process. Regaining continence can take as long as a year or two, and some patients fail to regain continence despite their best efforts.
- The rate of incontinence associated with a neobladder is estimated at 15% for male patients of any age, 10% to 15% for female patients under age 70, and 30% to 40% for female patients over age 70.
- It usually takes a few months or longer for a neobladder to stretch enough to store urine for 4 to 6 hours. While you are waiting for your neobladder to stretch, you will have to empty your neobladder every 2 hours.
- About 5% of male patients and up to 30% to 40% of female patients experience urinary retention with a neobladder. Patients who have urinary retention often require lifelong self-catheterization to empty their neobladder.
- All patients with a neobladder must learn self-catheterization in the event they have problems emptying their neobladder.
- A neobladder is a complex urinary tract reconstruction. It is a longer, more complex procedure than an ileal conduit, and requires a longer recovery time.

- Because a neobladder is a more complicated reconstructive procedure than an ileal conduit, it may require traveling a longer distance to find a surgeon who performs a high volume of this type of reconstruction.

- Previous treatment with radiation therapy in the pelvic or abdominal area(s) may disqualify you from having a neobladder.

- Because your surgeon may learn during the surgery that you are not a suitable candidate for a neobladder, it is important that you talk to your surgeon before the operation to discuss what type of reconstruction you want him or her to perform in the event that you cannot have a neobladder.

Continent Catheterizable Reservoir

A *continent catheterizable reservoir* is the third type of reconstruction (see figure 10.3). Like a neobladder, a continent catheterizable reservoir is called a *continent* urinary tract reconstruction because it stores urine inside the body.

How Does a Continent Catheterizable Reservoir Work?

Urine is produced in the kidneys and passes through the ureters — just as before the operation. From the ureters, urine flows into a newly created internal *pouch*, called a *continent catheterizable reservoir*, which stores urine. The continent catheterizable reservoir is connected at one end to the ureters and at the other end to a very small stoma (surgical opening) in the abdominal wall.

A catheter must be inserted into the stoma to drain urine from the pouch. This is called *catheterization*. The mechanism that allows for successful catheterization is usually a flap valve that permits the insertion of a catheter into the stoma to empty urine from the pouch and prevent urine from leaking between catheterizations.

At first, you will need to insert the catheter every 2 hours to keep the pouch from getting full and being subjected to undue stress. Over time, as the pouch heals, it will become stronger and increase in size, and you will be able to catheterize every 4 to 6 hours and remain dry in between. A small Band-Aid

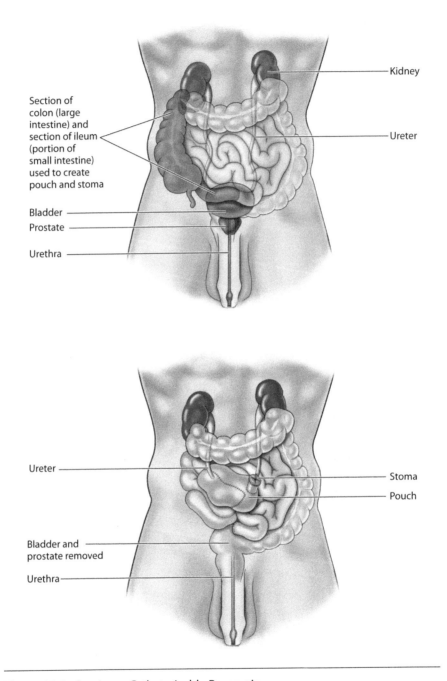

Figure 10.3 Continent Catheterizable Reservoir

can be used to cover the stoma when the stoma is not being used to empty the pouch. If you choose a continent catheterizable reservoir, your doctor or nurse will teach you how to insert a catheter into your stoma to empty the pouch.

How Is a Continent Catheterizable Reservoir Constructed?

To construct a continent catheterizable reservoir, the surgeon uses a section of the colon (large intestine) and a section of the ileum (a portion of the small intestine) to form an internal pouch. Next, the surgeon attaches the pouch to the ureters. Then the surgeon makes a very small opening, called a *stoma*, in the abdominal wall and connects the pouch to the stoma. The stoma is usually located in the umbilicus (also known as the belly button) to make it less noticeable on the body. The stoma created for this type of reconstruction is smaller than the one created for an ileal conduit. After constructing a continent catheterizable reservoir and stoma, the surgeon reattaches the remaining intestinal tract to permit normal digestion and bowel movements.

What Are the Risks and Complications Associated with a Continent Catheterizable Reservoir?

About 20% of patients with a continent catheterizable reservoir will require some form of corrective surgery or other intervention to repair or improve the function of their reconstruction. The most common problem associated with this type of reconstruction is a failure of the flap valve, which can result in urine leaking from the stoma. Other complications include scar formation, obstruction of the ureteral connections to the continent catheterizable reservoir, and chronic urinary tract infection.

Things to Consider About a Continent Catheterizable Reservoir

- Unlike patients with a neobladder, patients with a continent catheterizable reservoir do not empty urine through their urethra.
- A continent catheterizable reservoir is similar to an ileal conduit in that it requires a stoma — but unlike an ileal conduit, there is no need to wear an ostomy bag.

- A continent catheterizable reservoir must be drained every 4 to 6 hours by inserting a thin, flexible catheter (tube) into the stoma — called *catheterization.*

- A continent catheterizable reservoir is a complex urinary tract reconstruction. It is a longer, more complex procedure than an ileal conduit, and requires a longer recovery time.

- Because a continent catheterizable reservoir is a more complicated reconstructive procedure than an ileal conduit, it may require traveling a longer distance to find a surgeon who performs a high volume of this type of reconstruction.

- There is about a 20% chance that you will require corrective surgery or other type of intervention to repair or improve the function of your continent catheterizable reservoir.

Choosing a Surgeon

It is important that you ask your surgeon how many urinary tract reconstructions *of the type(s) you are considering* that he or she performs each year. Some surgeons perform mostly ileal conduit reconstructions, the most common and simplest form of urinary tract reconstruction. Other surgeons perform a high volume of neobladder and/or catheterizable reservoir reconstructions, which are more complex than an ileal conduit. Regardless of the type of urinary tract reconstruction you choose, it is in your best interest to find a surgeon who performs a high volume of the specific type of urinary tract reconstruction you will be undergoing.

Talking with Other Patients

While surgeons are very familiar with the operations they perform, they tend to be much less familiar with the personal experience of being a patient. Doctors tend to understand health care from a doctor's perspective. However, patients who have undergone a radical cystectomy have firsthand knowledge about what it is like to have this surgery and live with the urinary tract reconstruction they have chosen. It is often helpful to talk with patients who have had a radical cystectomy performed by your surgeon at the same medical center where you plan to have your surgery, particularly patients who have the same urinary tract reconstruction you are considering. Most doctors will be happy to give you the names of patients who are willing to talk to you.

CHAPTER 11

Recovery After a Radical Cystectomy

Patients who undergo a radical cystectomy often worry about how the surgery will affect their physical well-being, social functioning, and lifestyle in the days, months, and years after surgery. No matter what type of urinary tract reconstruction you choose, you will have to make significant adjustments after this life-changing surgery. Although the road to recovery is not without challenges, most people return to their normal activities within a few months of the operation. You may find it difficult to believe, but your life, with some adjustments, will gradually return to normal.

This chapter answers the following questions about life after a radical cystectomy:

- What is the hospital stay like after a radical cystectomy?
- What is recovery like when you get home?
- What follow-up care is needed after a radical cystectomy?
- What is the impact of a radical cystectomy on sexual function and fertility?
- For patients with an ileal conduit: What is involved in stoma care?

Your Postoperative Hospital Stay

After the operation is completed, you may be required to spend 24 hours in the intensive care unit for postoperative monitoring. However, not every hospital or surgeon requires the monitoring of patients in the intensive care unit after a radical cystectomy. This is often a matter of hospital and physician preference and is determined largely by the patient's overall condition and the outcome of the surgical procedure. If unanticipated complications such as significant bleeding or other problems occur during the operation, most doctors recommend postoperative monitoring in the intensive care unit for a period of time. Once the immediate postoperative period is over, you will be transferred to a regular room for the remainder of your hospital stay.

The following applies to all patients after a radical cystectomy, regardless of the type of urinary tract reconstruction they have.

Drains: When you wake up from the surgery, you will have one or two drains coming out of your abdomen adjacent to the incision made during your surgery. These drains are usually connected to vacuum reservoirs and serve to evacuate blood clots and remove excess fluid that accumulate in the vicinity of the incision immediately after surgery. These drains will be removed once your surgeon believes there is little risk of accumulating significant fluid in the area of the surgery. This usually occurs before you go home from the hospital.

Moving around/avoiding blood clots: The first day after your surgery, you will be expected to sit up in a chair and walk for brief periods. Walking can help to stimulate bowel function and promote healing in general. A physical therapist may come by to help you get started. Each day you will be asked to get out of bed and to gradually increase the amount of walking you do in the hall. You may also be asked to perform leg exercises. In addition, you will have white compression stockings, called *thrombo-embolic-deterrent (TED)* stockings, on your legs. You may also have a sleeve placed around each leg, called a *sequential compression device (SCD)*. These activities and devices reduce the risk of developing blood clots in your legs.

Caring for your lungs: Your nurse will show you how to do breathing exercises to reduce the risk of developing postoperative pneumonia. You will be taught how to use an incentive spirometer, a medical device that shows you how deeply you need to breathe in and out. These exercises will help re-expand your lungs and prevent fluid from building up in them.

Controlling pain: There are various ways of controlling postoperative pain, and you should use them. Many hospitals offer patient-controlled analgesia

(PCA), which allows patients to self-administer small doses of pain medication, as prescribed by their doctor. PCA uses a pump, which is attached to an IV line that is inserted into a vein. The pump can be pre-set to deliver a small, steady flow of pain medicine. In addition, the patient can increase the amount of pain medication, as needed, by pressing a button. Alternatively, the pump can be pre-set to deliver pain medicine only when the patient pushes the button. In either case, the total amount of pain medication is limited to an amount prescribed by the physician.

Getting back on solid foods: Your intestines, after having been manipulated during the surgery, usually slow down for a period of time. Your intestines have been traumatized, and it is very important to give them a chance to recover before it is time for them to go back to work digesting food. Gradually, during the first few days after your operation, your intestines will awaken and begin functioning again. At a rate of progress dictated by your intestines, you will gradually be introduced to solid foods until you can eat foods that approximate your diet before your surgery. You will be given ice chips at first, then move to clear liquids, then to soft foods, and then to solid foods. Once you are back on solid foods, you will be able to take medications orally.

How long you will be in the hospital: You can expect to be in the hospital for about 5 to 10 days after your surgery. One of the major factors that will determine when you are ready to go home is your intestinal activity. Your doctor will be looking for certain intestinal milestones. You must be able to eat a regular diet without getting nauseated and vomiting. You must also be able to move your bowels and pass gas. Exactly how long that takes will vary from patient to patient and will depend on several factors. Scar tissue from any prior abdominal surgery, the stress on your intestines during surgery, and the amount of pain medications you are taking all affect and slow down bowel activity. There may be internal swelling at the site where a piece of intestine was removed during urinary tract reconstruction. Until this swelling goes down, fluid may move through this area with some difficulty. All of these factors can combine to shut down intestinal activity temporarily, which usually starts to function normally again within a few days. Although you may feel that you are being held hostage by your intestines, moving (especially walking) can help stimulate bowel function and promote healing in general.

The following applies after a radical cystectomy, depending on the type of urinary tract reconstruction you have.

If you have a neobladder: As your neobladder is healing after surgery, you will have a catheter, often called a *Foley* catheter, passing through your urethra into your neobladder to drain urine. The catheter is connected to a drainage bag, which collects urine as it drains from the catheter. Most likely, the catheter will be removed during your initial postoperative visit about 3 weeks after surgery (discussed later in this chapter).

If you have a continent catheterizable reservoir: As your continent catheterizable reservoir is healing after surgery, you will have a catheter, referred to as a *stoma* catheter, passing through your stoma into your continent catheterizable reservoir to drain urine. In addition, as a safety precaution, you will have a larger catheter, called a *suprapubic* catheter, passing through your abdomen into your continent catheterizable reservoir to drain urine in the event that the stoma catheter becomes clogged. Both catheters are connected to drainage bags, which collect urine as it drains from the catheters. These catheters will not be removed at the time of your initial postoperative visit. Instead, they will be removed during subsequent follow-up visits, ranging from about 5 to 7 weeks after surgery (discussed later in this chapter).

If you have a neobladder or a continent catheterizable reservoir: Because neobladders and continent catheterizable reservoirs are made from intestinal tissue — and mucus is naturally produced by the intestines — you will have mucus in your urine if you have either of these urinary tract reconstructions. The mucus may become thick and block urine from draining through your catheter(s) — and thus must be cleared. While you are in the hospital, you will be taught how to flush (irrigate) sterile fluid through your catheter(s) to ensure that excess mucus does not accumulate and block the drainage of urine. It is important to understand that you will be responsible for flushing your catheter(s) when you get home.

If you have an ileal conduit: Unlike patients with a neobladder or a continent catheterizable reservoir, you will not have a catheter in place postoperatively. Instead, an external pouch, called an *ostomy bag*, will be attached with adhesive to the skin around your stoma before you leave the operating room. The ostomy bag collects urine as it drains from your stoma, preventing urine from leaking onto your skin. While you are in the hospital, an enterostomal therapy (ET) nurse will show you how to care for your stoma and change and empty your ostomy bag (discussed later in this chapter).

When You Get Home — the Road to Recovery

Leaving the hospital: Once your normal intestinal function has returned (passing gas and bowel movements), you are on a regular diet, your pain can be controlled with oral pain medication, and you are walking on your own, you will be discharged from the hospital. You will probably have a home health nurse for the first few days or weeks to check your surgical incision and make sure that you are caring for your catheter(s) and/or stoma properly.

Signs of infection: While you are in the hospital, you will have blood in your urine due to the surgery. However, by the time you leave the hospital, or within a few days thereafter, your urine should be clear of blood, although it may appear a bit cloudy because of mucus. Blood in your urine that is not related to trauma (for example, bumping your stoma) may be a sign of infection. Other signs of infection are a significant increase in the amount of mucus in your urine, a foul smell to your urine, fever, or pain in the kidney area. If you have any of these symptoms, you should call your doctor immediately.

Drinking fluids: It is important to drink plenty of fluids. The best way to prevent a urinary tract infection and the formation of kidney stones is to keep urine flowing through your urinary system. Unless your fluid intake is restricted for other reasons, make an effort to drink at least 6 to 8 glasses of liquid a day. When you get up in the morning, pour yourself a glass of water, juice, or milk (although water is best). As long as it is not alcohol, which dehydrates the body, the type of fluid you drink is not critical, unless you had kidney stones in the past and your doctor has adjusted your diet to help prevent kidney stone formation. You do not have to drink constantly, but it is good to keep on sipping several times an hour. Ideally, you should drink enough so that your urine is pale yellow in color. Darker urine is more concentrated and could be a sign that you are not sufficiently hydrated. If you have a neobladder or a continent catheterizable reservoir, drinking fluids will also help to dilute the mucus in your urine.

Weight loss: Most people lose from 10 to 25 pounds following surgery. Do not be concerned if you do not regain this weight quickly. If you are having problems with your appetite, be sure to talk to your doctor. Many things can affect your appetite, so the solution will be determined by the cause. Be sure to tell your doctor if food tastes metallic, salty, or tasteless, as these can be signs of a yeast infection in your mouth.

Bowel problems: Most people have diarrhea or constipation after a radical cystectomy because of the manipulation of the intestines during surgery. Usually these problems resolve within a few months after surgery. People with persistent bowel issues may require the care of a gastroenterologist, a physician who specializes in treating bowel disorders. For most people, bowel problems tend to resolve naturally with time. It is important to check with your surgeon before treating yourself, especially in the early weeks after surgery. Not all remedies are safe.

Diet: You will not have to make any dietary adjustments because of your surgery. However, in the first weeks after the operation, you may want to avoid hard-to-digest foods or high-fiber foods. Small quantities may be all right. It is a good idea to test the effects of small amounts before eating large quantities of these foods. Remember that you have had abdominal surgery and your body needs to re-adjust to the eating process.

Exercise: Exercise is an important part of the recovery process. It is very important to continue the walking you started in the hospital. Walking promotes healing and helps prevent the formation of blood clots, which can lead to a pulmonary embolism, a dangerous and potentially life-threatening condition. A pulmonary embolism can occur when blood clots that form in the veins of the legs or knees break off and travel to the lungs. A common sign of blood clots is pain in the lower legs or knees. Be sure to call your doctor immediately if you have any of these symptoms.

Lifting or straining: Although it is important to avoid heavy lifting or straining (do not lift more than 10 pounds) and to avoid any activities that could result in a blow to your abdomen, you can resume most of your preoperative activities within about 3 months of your surgery.

Lymphedema: You may develop lymphedema due to the removal of lymph nodes during your surgery. This is a condition in which extra lymph fluid builds in soft body tissues when lymphatic vessels are blocked or damaged. The main symptom of lymphedema is swelling in the legs or arms. Lymphedema usually develops within 3 years of the surgery, although it may develop many years later. Treatment for the symptoms of lymphedema may include medications and/or physical therapy.

Follow-up Care After a Radical Cystectomy

You will have your initial postoperative visit with your surgeon about 3 weeks after your surgery to check on your recovery.

If you have a neobladder, your Foley catheter will most likely be removed during your initial postoperative visit. After the catheter is removed, you will be taught how to empty your neobladder by urinating through your urethra. You will be instructed to urinate at regular intervals, the timing of which will be determined by your doctor. At this visit, you will also be taught *self-catheterization*, which requires that you insert a catheter through your urethra to empty urine from your neobladder. Self-catheterization will be necessary in the event you are unable to sufficiently empty your neobladder when urinating. It is likely that during this visit, your doctor will refer you to a physical therapist to help you gradually regain urinary continence.

If you have a continent catheterizable reservoir, your stoma catheter and suprapubic catheter will be left in place during your initial postoperative visit to allow for further healing. You will be asked to return for another visit about 2 weeks later (about 5 weeks after surgery). At this visit, your stoma catheter will be removed, and you will be taught how to *catheterize* (use a catheter to drain urine from) your continent catheterizable reservoir. As a precaution, the suprapubic catheter will be left in place while you are learning to catheterize. You will be asked to return for another visit about 2 weeks later (about 7 weeks after surgery) to have the suprapubic catheter removed, assuming you have learned to catheterize your continent catheterizable reservoir.

If you have an ileal conduit, during your initial postoperative visit, you should discuss any problems you are having with stoma care. Stoma care is discussed in detail at the end of this chapter.

Regardless of the type of urinary tract reconstruction you have, you will be asked to return for follow-up visits to monitor for recurrence of your disease. Follow-up tests and procedures include cystoscopies, imaging tests, and laboratory tests. During your follow-up care, your doctor will also monitor and/or treat any long-term or late treatment-related side effects.

Follow-up monitoring (surveillance) is a lifelong commitment. You will be asked to return for follow-up visits every 3 to 6 months for the first 2 years after surgery. After 2 years, if there is no evidence of disease, you will be asked to return every 6 months for the next 3 years for follow-up visits. If there is no evidence of disease after 5 years, you will be asked to return once a year for follow-up visits. After 5 years of being cancer free, the odds are good that the cancer will not return. Nevertheless, you will need to remain vigilant since late recurrences are known to occur.

Impact of a Radical Cystectomy on Sexual Function and Fertility

The following discusses the potential impact of a radical cystectomy on sexual function and fertility in men and women. It is important to understand that removing as much of the cancer as possible is usually the main goal of treatment, even if it has an adverse affect on sexual function and/or fertility.

Sexual Function

During a radical cystectomy, the prostate is removed in all men; and, in some women, it may be necessary to remove one or more reproductive organ(s). The removal of these organs has a wide-ranging effect on sexual functioning. The impact can be both physical and emotional, affecting both sexual activity and self-confidence.

The impact of a radical cystectomy on sexual function is usually age specific, with younger patients more likely to regain sexual function than older patients. In men, preoperative potency is also a major factor associated with recovering sexual function.

Patients who are sexually active should consult with their doctor before surgery to address any questions or concerns they have about potential changes in sexual function.

In Men

Because the prostate is attached to the bladder, and the prostate is a common site for the spread of bladder cancer in men, the prostate is always removed in male patients during a radical cystectomy. Removal of the prostate can result in difficulty having or maintaining an erection, called *erectile dysfunction* (*ED*). Because the nerves responsible for erections in men are located adjacent to the prostate, they are at risk of being damaged when the prostate is removed. These nerves may be able to be preserved if the surgeon performs a nerve-sparing radical cystectomy. This surgery results in preservation of full erectile function in approximately 60% of men age 50 or younger, 50% of men between the ages of 50 and 60, and 35% of men between the ages of 60 and 70. If erectile dysfunction occurs, it can often be treated with medications or, in some cases, with penile implants or other prosthetic devices. Removal of the prostate does not prevent men from having normal penile sensation, sexual drive, and achieving orgasm.

In Women

Women who undergo a radical cystectomy can experience sexual dysfunction, such as decreased orgasm, reduced vaginal lubrication, and difficulty with intercourse, particularly if during the surgery some or all of the woman's reproductive organs and associated nerves are removed.

The traditional operation for bladder removal in women has involved the complete removal of the uterus, cervix, ovaries, fallopian tubes, and a portion of the vagina. This extensive procedure was considered necessary because advanced stages of bladder cancer in women were thought to involve the female reproductive organs, such as the ovaries and uterus. However, contemporary studies performed in both the United States and Europe have shown that bladder cancer, even when invasive, rarely extends to these areas. Currently, surgeons try to spare as many organs and nerves associated with sexual function as possible when performing bladder removal surgery in women. As a result, sexual recovery in women after a radical cystectomy has improved significantly. Also, postoperative counseling related to sexual techniques and positions can make having sexual intercourse more comfortable for women.

Fertility

The following discusses the impact of a radical cystectomy on fertility (the ability to produce children) in men and women. Patients who want to have children after a radical cystectomy should talk to their doctor about the impact of the surgery on their fertility, and what measures they can take before the surgery to be able to produce children in the future.

In Men

After a radical cystectomy, men retain fertility but are unable to fertilize an egg through ejaculation. However, sperm can be aspirated from the testicles and used for artificial insemination.

Male patients who are planning to have a radical cystectomy and wish to have children in the future should consider banking their sperm before their surgery.

In Women

In women, infertility after a radical cystectomy results from the removal of the uterus and other sexual organs during the surgery. Female patients who are planning to have a radical cystectomy and want to have children in the future should ask their doctor whether the surgery will potentially involve the removal of any of their reproductive organs — and, if so, the impact this will have on their ability to have children.

A WORD TO THE PARTNER

You may feel that you are going through many of the same adjustments your loved one is experiencing after a radical cystectomy. In fact, you are. You will certainly ride the same emotional roller coaster and worry about the same things. Do not underestimate or ignore your needs at this time. Though you are concerned about your partner, be sure to allow time for yourself — stop, have lunch with a friend, recharge your batteries. Your partner's road to recovery following a radical cystectomy is going to feel more like a marathon than a sprint. You need to take care of yourself in order to have the energy and emotional stamina needed to support your partner during this journey.

Although many people try to do everything for the person who is recovering, you may find this is not the best approach for your own or your partner's mental health. The key to your partner rebuilding his or her self-esteem is for him or her to return as quickly as possible to the level of self-care and independence enjoyed prior to the illness. Self-care is important as a way of feeling that things are returning to the usual or normal pattern.

While there is no denying that a radical cystectomy is a life-changing surgery, your understanding and support for your partner will be an important part of the healing process. Open communication between you and your partner will help both of you cope with the physical and emotional adjustments that will be required during recovery.

For Patients with an Ileal Conduit:
Caring for Your Stoma

The remainder of this chapter addresses the challenges faced by patients as they learn to care for and adapt to living with an ileal conduit.

During Your Hospital Stay

After the operation, while you are still in the hospital, there will be many things to learn about caring for your stoma. Although your ET nurse will help guide the process, you will have primary responsibility for the pace of your learning. You may feel that you need a day or two before you are ready to take on the task of learning stoma care — or you may be anxious to get started. In either case, the teaching and learning process will proceed in small steps tailored to meet your individual needs.

The first bridge to cross is looking at your stoma for the first time. The ostomy bag that was attached while you were in the operating room is usually changed one or two days after the surgery. This will be your first opportunity to see your stoma. Most people react to seeing their stoma by saying it is bigger than they thought it would be. It is important to understand that a stoma is usually swollen at first and will shrink to its final size by about 4 to 6 weeks following surgery. The timing and amount of change varies from person to person. The size of your stoma may not change at all, or it may shrink to half its original size. When you touch your stoma, you will notice that you feel no sensation from it, even though it may look like it is sore and tender.

Before you leave the hospital, your ET nurse will show you how to change and empty your ostomy bag. After you remove the ostomy bag, you will have to clean the skin around your stoma, called the *peristomal* area. This is done by simply washing the area with soap and water, rinsing it well, and patting it dry. It is a good idea to avoid highly perfumed or very creamy soaps because they may cause itching or interfere with the adhesive seal on the ostomy bag. People with extremely sensitive skin may choose to wash with water only. For these people, the peristomal area may be coated with a liquid skin barrier or protector and allowed to dry. Occasionally, particularly as you are learning to change your ostomy bag, you may develop irritation of the skin or stoma. You should work with your ET nurse to resolve this problem.

You will then prepare the ostomy bag to fit around your stoma. Your stoma should be measured to be sure the ostomy bag has the proper-sized opening. If necessary, the bag will need to be cut to fit around your stoma, without allowing any skin to be exposed to urine. Once the size of your stoma has stabilized, pre-cut ostomy bags are available for those who do not want to bother cutting the opening each time. Many people cut the opening in their ostomy bag while their stoma is changing size, and then switch to pre-cut bags once their stoma shrinks to its final size.

When You Get Home

For anyone who has an ileal conduit reconstruction, emptying their ostomy bag becomes an ongoing part of daily life. Whether you are at home, at work, or at a party, you will need to empty your ostomy bag at least 3 or 4 times during an average day. Since it is always important to drink fluids — at least 6 to 8 glasses of water a day are recommended unless your liquids are restricted for other reasons — the timing will be partially dependent on how much you have had to drink.

You will have to make a decision about how you want to empty your ostomy bag overnight. Your kidneys usually produce more urine during the night than your regular ostomy bag can hold. You will have two nighttime options — get up at least once a night to empty your regular ostomy bag or attach your regular ostomy bag to an extension drainage tube that is connected to a larger night bag. This allows your regular ostomy bag to drain into the larger night bag throughout the night. The night bag can be emptied in the morning. The advantage of using a night bag is that it allows you to sleep throughout the night.

Ostomy bags must be changed every 3 to 4 days. Wearing an ostomy bag longer than that can lead to a urinary tract infection due to bacteria that grows in the bag over time. After you have become familiar with the process, changing your ostomy bag will take only a few minutes. You may wish to combine the task with showering. Although you may develop a twice-a-week routine for changing your ostomy bag, most people carry back-up supplies with them for unexpected situations. It is always a good idea to keep an extra ostomy bag with you just in case.

Ostomy bags are made so they are not noticeable under clothing. They are held to the skin with strong, hypoallergenic adhesives that hold up through normal showering, bathing, exercise, or swimming. Virtually all ostomy bags manufactured today have anti-reflux valves or separate compartments that keep urine in the lower part of the bag from flowing backward into the stoma and toward the kidney. Both clear and opaque ostomy bags are available. They come in a variety of shapes and textures and with a variety of adhesives. Two-piece ostomy bags are also available, with the sticky portion and the collecting portion separated to allow the size and shape of the bag to be changed without removing the adhesive from the skin. Some people like to wear a larger, clear ostomy bag most of the time and switch to a smaller or opaque bag during physical activity such as exercise or sexual intercourse. Many attractive under-garments are available that cover the ostomy bag during intimate moments. You will be able to select a reliable, comfortable ostomy bag that meets your needs.

If you encounter any problems with stoma care, you should contact your ET nurse for help in resolving your issues.

Many patients find it helpful to talk with other patients who, like themselves, are living with a stoma. The United Ostomy Associations of America, Inc., (UOAA) is an association of more than 340 UOAA-affiliated support groups dedicated to improving the quality of life for people with an ostomy. You can locate a UOAA-affiliated support group closest to your area by going to the UOAA website at *www.ostomy.org*.

Living with an Ileal Conduit

As you look ahead to living with an ileal conduit, it is natural to have concerns about how it will affect your social relationships and activities. In addition to fears about changes in your appearance, the thought of the loss of urinary control is frightening to many people. Learning self-care is the quickest way to gain a sense of control. In the days following your surgery and during your recovery at home, as you become more and more competent at the tasks neces-sary for stoma care, your fears will subside and you will gain a greater sense of control of your bodily functions.

Many people experience an emotional letdown after they get home from the hospital. Activities like taking walks (malls are great for this in bad weather) or going out to dinner or the movies are important steps in adjusting to life with an ileal conduit. At first, you may feel you have to force yourself to get out and do something, because you feel self-conscious about wearing an ostomy bag. Sometimes the only way to convince yourself that you are okay and that you can feel comfortable socializing with others is to go ahead and mingle with other people. You will be amazed at how oblivious others can be to changes that seem major to you.

CHAPTER 12

Bladder Preservation Therapy

Bladder preservation therapy is a treatment option for selected patients with muscle-invasive bladder cancer. This approach, also known as *bladder-sparing therapy* or *trimodality therapy (TMT)*, treats bladder cancer without removing the bladder.

Bladder preservation therapy combines three treatment modalities (methods) — a *TURBT*, *systemic chemotherapy*, and *radiation therapy*. After the removal of all visible cancer with a TURBT (transurethral resection of bladder tumor), systemic chemotherapy and radiation are given concurrently. The combination of systemic chemotherapy and radiation is called *chemoradiation*.

This chapter answers the following questions about bladder preservation therapy:

- Who is a good candidate for bladder preservation therapy?
- What is involved in the decision to have bladder preservation therapy?
- What is the treatment for bladder preservation therapy?
- What is the follow-up care after bladder preservation therapy?
- What are the side effects of bladder preservation therapy?

Who Is a Good Candidate for Bladder Preservation Therapy?

The careful selection of patients for bladder preservation therapy is key to achieving good outcomes with this approach. To determine if you are a good candidate for bladder preservation therapy, you will need to be evaluated by a urologic oncologist, preferably at a cancer center with experience and expertise in bladder preservation therapy. A thorough evaluation will include a complete medical history; a physical examination; blood tests; a TURBT; a CT or MRI scan of the chest, abdomen, and pelvis; and a bone scan.

The following discusses the factors doctors must consider to determine whether a person with bladder cancer is a good candidate for bladder preservation therapy.

Tumor Stage

The *stage* of your tumor is a key factor in determining if you are a good candidate for bladder preservation therapy. Patients with stage T2 or stage T3a bladder cancer are considered better candidates for bladder preservation therapy than patients with stage T3b or stage T4a disease. The lower the stage of your tumor, the more likely that all visible cancer can be removed during a TURBT and that the disease is confined to the bladder.

Patients with bladder cancer that has metastasized (spread) outside the bladder to surrounding lymph nodes and/or distant sites are *not* good candidates for bladder preservation therapy. These patients are usually treated with systemic chemotherapy (discussed in chapter 13).

As mentioned earlier, bladder preservation therapy is a treatment option for selected patients with muscle-invasive bladder cancer (stages T2–T4a). However, it may also be an option for patients with high-grade, stage T1 non-muscle-invasive bladder cancer who do not respond to standard therapies for non-muscle-invasive disease.

Ability to Have a Complete TURBT

One of the most important factors in determining whether you are a good candidate for bladder preservation therapy is the extent to which your tumor can be surgically removed (resected) during a TURBT. The goal of a TURBT during bladder preservation therapy is to remove *all* visible bladder cancer. This is called a *complete* TURBT.

Patients with earlier-stage tumors are more likely to have a complete (or almost complete) TURBT, which puts them in a better position to succeed with the next phase of bladder preservation therapy — chemoradiation. The more complete the TURBT, the more likely that chemoradiation will be effective in eradicating any remaining (residual) bladder cancer.

Number and Size of Tumor(s)

You are more likely to succeed with bladder preservation therapy if you have a *single* (solitary) tumor as opposed to multiple tumors. In addition, you are more likely to succeed with bladder preservation therapy if the *size* of your tumor is less than 5 centimeters (cm).

Location of Tumor(s)

The *location* of your tumor(s) is an important factor in determining whether you are a good candidate for a bladder-preserving approach. An important predictor of success during bladder preservation therapy is the ability to remove all visible cancer during a TURBT. For all visible disease to be removed, the tumor must be located in a part of the bladder that allows the doctor to both see and reach the disease. Tumors located in the right lateral wall, left lateral wall, or lower anterior wall are well situated for bladder preservation therapy. Tumors in these locations can more easily be seen and removed than tumors in other parts of the bladder.

In addition to being visible and accessible, the tumor must be situated such that the radiation administered during bladder preservation therapy will not impair the ability of the bladder and/or surrounding organs to function properly. For example, a tumor located in the dome of the bladder may not be suitable for bladder preservation therapy, because the tumor may be too close to the small intestine, which can be damaged by radiation therapy.

No CIS (Carcinoma In Situ)

A patient with CIS is *not* a good candidate for bladder preservation therapy. Radiation therapy (an important component of bladder preservation therapy) is not an effective treatment for CIS. Patients with CIS are better served with a radical cystectomy.

No Hydronephrosis

A tumor located at or near the opening of the ureter to the bladder can cause the ureter to become obstructed — leading to *hydronephrosis,* a backup of urine into the kidneys that causes the kidneys to swell. Patients with hydronephrosis do *not* do well with bladder preservation therapy and are better served with a radical cystectomy.

Kidney Function

A good candidate for bladder preservation therapy must have *good kidney function,* which is required for treatment with cisplatin, a chemotherapy drug used during chemoradiation.

Bladder Function

To be a good candidate for bladder preservation therapy, you must have a *well-functioning bladder.* Unless you have a well-functioning bladder at the conclusion of therapy, there is no reason to undergo bladder preservation therapy.

Age and General Health

Generally, the younger you are and the better your general health, the more likely that you are a good candidate for this approach. Patients with certain co-existing medical conditions and/or treatment histories — such as inflammatory bowel disease, prior surgery in the pelvis, or previous radiation therapy in the pelvis — may be less suited for bladder preservation therapy.

Diagnosed with Urothelial Cell Carcinoma

Most studies investigating the use of bladder preservation therapy have involved patients with *urothelial cell carcinoma,* which accounts for about 90% of all patients with bladder cancer. There is limited research to support the use of bladder preservation therapy in patients with *non-urothelial* bladder cancer, such as squamous cell carcinoma. The prevailing view is that patients with non-urothelial bladder cancer are better served with a radical cystectomy.

Selection Criteria for Bladder Preservation Therapy

Patients best suited for bladder preservation therapy are those with the following:

- Stage T2 bladder cancer
- No evidence of metastatic bladder cancer
- All visible tumor removed during TURBT (*complete* TURBT)
- Single (solitary) tumor less than 5 centimeters (cm)
- Tumors located in right lateral wall, left lateral wall, or lower anterior wall
- No CIS
- No hydronephrosis
- Good kidney function
- Good bladder function
- Good general health
- Diagnosed with urothelial cell carcinoma

To determine if you are a good candidate for bladder preservaton therapy, you need to be evaluated by a urologic oncologist, preferably at a cancer center that treats a high volume of patients with bladder preservation therapy.

The Decision to Have Bladder Preservation Therapy

If your doctor determines that you are a good candidate for bladder preservation therapy, you will have to decide whether this approach is right for you. A radical cystectomy is the standard treatment for muscle-invasive bladder cancer against which all other treatment options must be measured.

Bladder preservation therapy should only be undertaken when the likelihood of achieving a cure without removing the bladder is equivalent to the likelihood of achieving a cure with bladder removal surgery (radical cystectomy) — *and* there is a high likelihood that satisfactory bladder function can be preserved when retaining the bladder. Keeping your bladder will not be worthwhile if it does not function properly.

If after carefully considering the likely outcomes of your treatment options, you are comfortable that the likelihood of a cure with bladder preservation therapy is the same as with a radical cystectomy, and that your bladder will function well, it is important to consider the following additional factors before making a final decision.

Requires Treatment at a Cancer Center with Expertise in Bladder Preservation Therapy

Bladder preservation therapy is a highly specialized, multidisciplinary approach, requiring the close cooperation of multiple specialists. If you are considering bladder preservation therapy, it is important to be evaluated and treated by a team of specialists who have expertise in bladder preservation therapy and who treat a high volume of patients with this approach.

Bladder Preservation Therapy Is Emotionally and Physically Demanding

Bladder preservation therapy takes several months. It is demanding emotionally and physically both in terms of the time it takes and the toll it can take on the body. To fully understand all aspects of your protocol, you should meet with the urologic oncologist who will be performing the TURBT, the medical oncologist who will be administering the chemotherapy, and the radiation oncologist who will be administering the radiation therapy. Bladder preservation therapy requires a motivated patient — someone with a strong commitment and a willingness to accept the emotional and physical demands of this treatment approach.

May Need a Radical Cystectomy if Bladder Preservation Therapy Fails

If bladder preservation therapy fails to eradicate your disease, you will likely be offered a radical cystectomy, called a *salvage* radical cystectomy. If you undergo a radical cystectomy after bladder preservation therapy, your previous treatment with radiation may impact your options for urinary tract reconstruction. Because the intestines can be damaged by radiation during bladder preservation therapy, you may not be a candidate for a neobladder. Instead, you would likely be offered an ileal conduit. If you are considering bladder preservation therapy, be sure to ask your physician about the potential impact of radiation on your options for urinary tract reconstruction in the event that you later need a radical cystectomy.

> You must always keep in mind that curing your cancer is more important than preserving your bladder. The main objective is to save your life. Having your native bladder is nice, but you can have a good life without your native bladder. In fact, many people do.

Bladder Preservation Therapy: A Three-Pronged Approach

Bladder preservation therapy is a *trimodal* approach, which means it combines *three* treatment modalities (methods). Bladder preservation begins with a TURBT, followed by chemoradiation (systemic chemotherapy and radiation). This treatment requires a multidisciplinary approach, in which the urologic oncologist works in cooperation with the medical oncologist (a doctor who specializes in using systemic chemotherapy to treat cancer) and the radiation oncologist (a doctor who specializes in using radiation to treat cancer).

It should be noted that protocols (treatment plans) for bladder preservation therapy are continually evolving as doctors investigate the best ways to administer this therapy — and protocols may vary somewhat from cancer center to cancer center. Be sure to ask your doctor for a description of the specific bladder preservation protocol that is being recommended for you.

TURBT

Assuming you have met the selection criteria for bladder preservation therapy, and you have decided that this approach is right for you, the next step is for your urologic oncologist to perform a **TURBT**. The purpose of the TURBT is to make sure that the resection (removal) of the bladder tumor is as complete and thorough as possible.

If after your TURBT your urologic oncologist determines that the cancer has been maximally removed, you will proceed with the next phase of bladder preservation therapy — chemoradiation.

Chemoradiation

Even when all visible cancer is removed during a TURBT, cancer cells may still be present. Therefore, the next step in bladder preservation therapy is **chemoradiation**.

The initial phase of chemoradiation is called the **induction phase**. During this phase, systemic chemotherapy (administered by a medical oncologist) and radiation therapy (administered by a radiation oncologist) are given concurrently, with the goal of killing any remaining cancer cells.

During the induction phase of chemoradiation, systemic chemotherapy (cancer drugs delivered intravenously) serves two purposes. First, systemic chemotherapy is used to kill cancer cells in the bladder and elsewhere in the body. Second, when given before radiation therapy, systemic chemotherapy can make cancer cells more likely to respond to radiation (called *radiosensitization*).

Unlike systemic chemotherapy, which treats the entire body, radiation treats cancer cells in specific treatment areas, called *treatment fields* or *radiation fields*. During the induction phase of chemoradiation, radiation is directed at cancer cells inside and immediately outside the bladder, as well as in nearby lymph nodes, which can also harbor cancer cells. The goal of radiation is to kill cancer cells while at the same time preserving normal bladder function. Too much radiation can damage the bladder, as well as the nearby colon and rectum. Not enough radiation can limit its effectiveness in destroying cancer cells.

After the completion of the induction phase — followed by a break of about 3 weeks to rest and recover — you will be evaluated to determine your response. This evaluation usually includes a cystoscopy, urine cytology, and imaging test(s), as well as another TURBT to obtain biopsies from the original tumor site(s). If you have achieved a *complete response* — meaning there is no evidence of disease — you will proceed to the next phase of chemoradiation, called the **consolidation phase**. If you have *not* achieved a complete response to the induction phase, you will not proceed to the consolidation phase. Instead, you will be offered a different treatment based on the stage of your disease — most likely a salvage radical cystectomy, which may be followed by additional systemic chemotherapy.

The consolidation phase of chemoradiation consists of systemic chemotherapy and radiation given concurrently, which may or may not be followed by systemic chemotherapy given alone. After completion of the consolidation phase — followed by a break of about 6 to 8 weeks — you will be evaluated again to determine your response. If there is no evidence of cancer (that is, if you continue to have a complete response), you can proceed to follow-up care and surveillance. However, if after completing the consolidation phase, there is evidence of cancer, you will be offered a different treatment based on the stage of your disease — most likely a salvage radical cystectomy, which may be followed by additional systemic chemotherapy.

Follow-up Care After Bladder Preservation Therapy

After completing bladder preservation therapy, you will need to return for periodic follow-up visits with your urologic oncologist to monitor for a recurrence (return) of your cancer. Regular follow-up monitoring, called *surveillance*, is essential, so that any sign of a recurrence of cancer can be treated as early as possible. These visits may include a physical examination, cystoscopy, and urine cytology. In addition, you will have regularly scheduled TURBTs to obtain biopsies, and CT or MRI scans. During your follow-up care, your doctor will also monitor and/or treat any long-term or late treatment-related side effects.

For the first 2 years after treatment, you will need to return for follow-up visits every 3 to 4 months. After 2 years, if there is no evidence of cancer, you will need to return for follow-up visits every 6 months for the next 3 years. After 5 years, if there is no evidence of disease, the odds are good that the cancer will not return. Nevertheless, you will need annual follow-up visits since late recurrences are known to occur. Surveillance after bladder preservation therapy is a lifelong commitment. If you have a recurrence of your disease during surveillance, you will be offered treatment option(s) based on the stage of your disease.

What Are the Side Effects of Bladder Preservation Therapy?

Potential side effects and risks associated with a TURBT are bleeding, pain and/or burning during urination, urinary tract infection, and bladder perforation. Most side effects resolve soon after treatment.

Potential short-term side effects of chemoradiation include a decrease in blood cell counts, fatigue, diarrhea, nausea, vomiting, and bladder irritation. Medications are available to treat most of these side effects, which usually resolve soon after treatment.

Potential long-term or late side effects of chemoradiation include neuropathy (numbness in the feet), early menopause in women, impotence in men (depending on the age and pre-treatment potency status of the male patient), a poorly functioning bladder, and occasional rectal bleeding or bowel urgency. In addition, radiation therapy can cause scar tissue in the treated areas, and can complicate or prevent future surgery in areas of the body previously treated with radiation.

Part 4 consists of **Chapter 13**, which discusses *metastatic bladder cancer* and how it is treated. Metastatic bladder cancer is the most advanced form of bladder cancer and the most difficult to treat. About 5% of bladder cancer is metastatic at the time of diagnosis.

CHAPTER 13

Metastatic Bladder Cancer

The spread of bladder cancer outside the bladder to surrounding lymph nodes and/or distant sites, such as the lung, liver, or bone, is called **metastatic** bladder cancer. Systemic chemotherapy is the primary treatment (treatment given initially) for metastatic bladder cancer.

This chapter answers the following questions about metastatic bladder cancer:

- How is metastatic bladder cancer diagnosed?
- What is the staging system for metastatic bladder cancer?
- What you need to know about systemic chemotherapy
- Immunotherapy as a treatment for metastatic bladder cancer
- Are clinical trials a treatment option for metastatic bladder cancer?
- When is radiation therapy used?
- What is palliative care?

How Is Metastatic Bladder Cancer Diagnosed?

In most patients, the spread of bladder cancer to lymph nodes and/or distant sites can be detected by imaging tests, such as a CT scan or an MRI. In some patients, however, there may be hidden (occult) metastatic disease that is too small to be detected by imaging tests. These tiny tumors, called *micrometastases,* can be diagnosed only after tissue is removed surgically and examined under a microscope.

What Is the Staging System for Metastatic Bladder Cancer?

The system for staging bladder cancer is called the ***TNM staging system***, which combines the initials T (primary tumor), N (lymph node), and M (distant metastasis) to indicate the depth and extent of the disease. In this system, the initials N and M are used to stage metastatic bladder cancer. The initial **N** indicates the absence or presence of lymph node involvement, and the initial **M** indicates the absence or presence of distant metastasis.

The following shows how the initials N and M are used in the TNM staging system to classify metastatic bladder cancer:

N0: No cancer is present in lymph node(s).

N1: Cancer is present in one lymph node near the bladder.

N2: Cancer is present in more than one lymph node near the bladder.

N3: Cancer is present in lymph nodes located at some distance from the bladder.

M0: There is no evidence of distant metastasis.

M1: There is evidence of distant metastasis.

The higher the stage of the primary tumor (T), the more likely that metastasis will occur.

There is a subcategory of stage T4 bladder cancer — called ***T4b*** — that is treated like metastatic disease, even when there is no evidence of lymph node involvement or distant metastasis. Stage T4b disease involves the rectum, pelvic wall, or abdominal wall — and, as such, cannot be removed surgically. Therefore, stage T4b is categorized and treated as metastatic disease.

For a more in-depth discussion of the TNM staging system, see chapter 5.

What You Need to Know About Systemic Chemotherapy

Systemic chemotherapy is the primary treatment for metastatic bladder cancer. Given intravenously (into a vein), systemic chemotherapy enters the bloodstream and kills cancer cells throughout the body. The use of systemic chemotherapy can sometimes extend the lives of patients for many years and, for some patients, may be curative.

This section answers the following questions about the use of systemic chemotherapy in treating metastatic bladder cancer:

- How does systemic chemotherapy work?
- What type of medical specialist do you need for systemic chemotherapy?
- What chemotherapy drugs are used to treat metastatic bladder cancer?
- What is the course of treatment with systemic chemotherapy?
- What are the side effects of systemic chemotherapy?
- Will you be able to work during systemic chemotherapy?
- How will you be monitored after systemic chemotherapy ends?

How Does Systemic Chemotherapy Work?

Normal bladder cells grow and divide in an orderly fashion. On the other hand, bladder cancer cells are characterized by uncontrolled growth and proliferation and may have the capacity to metastasize (spread) to other parts of the body.

Chemotherapy drugs eradicate cancer cells by stopping the ability of cancer cells to grow and divide. For cell growth to occur, a cell must constantly duplicate its DNA, the genetic material in cells, and pass the DNA on to its offspring cells through cell division. Certain chemotherapy drugs are designed to attack DNA so that the offspring cells receive ineffective copies of the genetic material needed by the cells to survive. Other drugs interfere with the proper functioning of cell division. And other drugs inhibit pathways needed for cancer cell survival and/or proliferation, thereby ultimately causing the death of cancer cells. All of these drugs have the goal of killing cancer cells or making it harder for cancer cells to survive, proliferate, and/or spread.

What Type of Medical Specialist Do You Need for Systemic Chemotherapy?

Initially, you will consult with a urologist or urologic oncologist to make a diagnosis. If there is evidence of metastatic disease, you will be referred to a medical oncologist, a doctor who specializes in using systemic chemotherapy drugs to treat cancer.

Your medical oncologist will be responsible for determining the most appropriate chemotherapy *treatment plan* (also called *regimen* or *protocol*), administering the chemotherapy, and monitoring your treatment response and any adverse side effects. It is important to select a medical oncologist who is experienced in treating bladder cancer.

Before beginning systemic chemotherapy, you will undergo comprehensive testing to determine the best treatment plan for you. The evaluation will include testing your kidney, liver, and heart — and will consider where the cancer has spread, your age, and your general health.

On your first visit to your medical oncologist, you are likely to feel anxious and fearful of what lies ahead. It is important to prepare for the consultation with your medical oncologist. Write down your questions and concerns beforehand, and ask all of your questions. No question is a stupid question. If you do not get an answer, or you do not understand the answer, it is important to keep asking until you do.

Questions to Ask Your Medical Oncologist When Choosing a Treatment Plan

The following are questions to ask your medical oncologist when choosing a treatment plan:

- What are my treatment options?
- What are the benefits and goals of each option, and how will response be measured?
- What are the potential side effects of each option, including short-term, long-term, and late effects?
- Is participating in a clinical trial a possible option?
- What treatment plan do you recommend, and why?

Because there may be different opinions about the best treatment plan, you may want to get a second opinion from another medical oncologist. After consulting with your medical oncologist and possibly getting a second opinion, and with the support of family members and/or friends, you will be better prepared to make an informed decision about the treatment plan that is best for you.

What Chemotherapy Drugs Are Used to Treat Metastatic Bladder Cancer?

Platinum-based (including cisplatin) chemotherapy regimens are primary treatments for metastatic bladder cancer. The older regimen, called *MVAC*, uses a combination of four chemotherapy drugs: methotrexate, vinblastine, doxorubicin (Adriamycin), and cisplatin. A newer regimen, called *GC*, uses a combination of gemcitabine and cisplatin. MVAC and GC have produced comparable response rates in patients with metastatic bladder cancer. However, since GC has proved to be less toxic and better tolerated than MVAC, GC has become an accepted alternative to MVAC.

Although platinum-based chemotherapy regimens are generally the primary treatments for patients with metastatic bladder cancer, they are not suitable for patients with poor kidney function. A chemotherapy drug called *carboplatin* is often used as a substitute for cisplatin for treating patients with insufficient kidney function.

HOW IS RESPONSE TO SYSTEMIC CHEMOTHERAPY MEASURED?

You will come across unfamiliar terms related to systemic chemotherapy, including terms that describe how a patient's response is measured. The following terminology is used to describe the outcomes of systemic chemotherapy.

Cure: No evidence of cancer for at least 5 years. A cure is no guarantee that the cancer will not return, but people who are cancer-free for 5 years or longer are much less likely to have a recurrence of their disease.

Response: An improvement as a result of treatment, such as a decrease in the size of the tumor.

Complete response (also called *complete remission*): No evidence of disease, but not necessarily a cure, since there may be microscopic cancer cells left behind that are too small to be detected by imaging tests. Although a complete response is not the same as a cure, there cannot be a cure without a complete response.

Partial response (also called *partial remission*): A decrease in the total amount of disease by more than 50%.

Response rate: The percentage of patients whose cancer improves as a result of treatment.

Stable disease: No major change in the size of the tumor. Tumors can change by 25% — either growing or shrinking — and still be considered stable.

Disease progression: The tumor has advanced to a higher stage and/or grade.

What Is the Course of Treatment with Systemic Chemotherapy?

Systemic chemotherapy for bladder cancer is typically given over a course of 3 to 6 months, but can be given for a longer or shorter period of time. *Treatment cycles* are repeated on a regular schedule with periods of rest in between. The course of treatment is likely to consist of 4 to 8 treatment cycles, with each cycle lasting about 2 to 3 weeks. A treatment cycle includes the time during which you are receiving therapy and the time until your next cycle, which allows time for your body to recover. Your treatment during each cycle will last from a few hours to a few days, depending on the drug or combination of drugs you are receiving.

Before each treatment cycle, you will have blood tests to determine if you can proceed with the next treatment cycle. The blood tests will check to see how well your kidneys are working, and check your red blood cell, white blood cell, and blood platelet counts. Low blood counts can result in side effects such as infection, fatigue, bruising, and bleeding. If you have a low blood count, your treatment may be delayed for a week or so, or you may be given a lower drug dose.

What Are the Side Effects of Systemic Chemotherapy?

Chemotherapy drugs work by killing cancer cells, but they can also damage normal, healthy cells as well. Damage to healthy cells as a result of chemotherapy causes *side effects,* which can occur in different body systems, at different times, in varying durations, and with differing amounts of intensity.

There are potential short-term (acute), long-term (chronic), and late side effects of systemic chemotherapy. *Short-term* side effects start shortly after the administration of therapy and usually taper off by the end of each treatment cycle. *Long-term* side effects begin shortly after the administration of therapy and can continue for months or years after the completion of treatment. *Late* side effects occur months or years after treatment ends.

Short-term side effects of systemic chemotherapy may include fatigue, weakness, nausea, headaches, dizziness, vomiting, loss of appetite, weight loss, hair loss, infection, fever, bruising, bleeding, shortness of breath, chest pain, increase in heart rate, and diarrhea. Some of these side effects are due to a reduction in blood counts, which is common during systemic chemotherapy. For example, low red blood cell count (anemia) can result in fatigue, weakness, shortness of breath, headaches, dizziness, chest pain, or an increase in heart rate. Low white blood cell count increases the risk of infection. Low blood platelet count increases the risk of bruising and risk of bleeding from the nose, gums, and rectum.

Your blood counts will be monitored on a regular basis during the course of treatment. Be sure to discuss with your doctor how to manage the side effects of low blood counts, and symptoms to watch for that require immediate medical attention. For example, if your white blood cell count drops below a certain level and you have a fever with temperature above 100.4°F, you would need to be hospitalized and given intravenous antibiotics to prevent a serious infection.

There are medications to prevent and control many of the short-term side effects of systemic chemotherapy. Once you have gone through a cycle or two of systemic chemotherapy, you will become more knowledgeable about how well you tolerate the therapy and what you can and cannot do during the course of treatment. If side effects persist, this may suggest to your doctor that a change in therapy or a change in dose or drug is needed.

Long-term side effects of systemic chemotherapy may include anemia (low red blood cell count), sterility, infertility, and nerve damage. Anemia will usually resolve over time, but you may need blood transfusions or growth factor injections to help restore your red blood cell count. For some patients, infertility is a concern. Men may want to consider banking their sperm if they want the option of fathering children after treatment. Women who want the option of having children after treatment should consult with their gynecologist about side effects of chemotherapy related to fertility. Women's menstrual periods may become irregular or cease altogether. Chemotherapy can have effects on unborn children, so adequate birth control, if appropriate, is needed while receiving therapy. If a woman becomes pregnant during therapy, she should talk with her doctor about the implications and discuss how to move forward. Nerve damage, called *neuropathy*, is another possible side effect.

Improvements in the management of side effects have eased the burden on patients as they undergo systemic chemotherapy. Supportive care during treatment includes medications to prevent and control side effects and to ensure the optimal delivery of therapy at its planned dosages and schedules. In order to achieve optimal outcomes from treatment and maximize quality of life, it is imperative to manage the side effects of treatment.

Late side effects refer to conditions that appear many months or years after the completion of treatment. Potential late side effects of systemic chemotherapy include *second cancers*, which refer to the development of different primary cancers elsewhere in the body. Fortunately, the onset of second cancers as a result of chemotherapy is rare, occurring in less than 2% of patients.

Will You Be Able to Work During Systemic Chemotherapy?

You may have questions about your ability to work during systemic chemotherapy. Because the side effects of chemotherapy drugs differ from person to person, you will not be able to predict the impact of chemotherapy on your ability to work until after you have begun therapy.

Depending on your treatment plan, you may be able to return to work the same day as your treatment. Other regimens can take most of the day to administer, and others may require hospitalization. You will have to adjust your work schedule to accommodate your particular situation.

How Will You Be Monitored After Systemic Chemotherapy?

After you have completed treatment, your doctor will recommend a schedule of follow-up visits and surveillance tests, such as imaging tests, cystoscopy, and/or urine cytology, to monitor for disease recurrence and/or progression. Your doctor will also monitor any long-term or late side effects. If you have new or recurring symptoms or side effects between scheduled follow-up visits, be sure to call your doctor.

If your cancer recurs, you may need additional tests to determine the location and extent of your disease. Based on this information, your doctor will explain your treatment options. When considering your treatment options, ask your doctor if a clinical trial is a possible option.

A fear of cancer recurrence is common among bladder cancer survivors. If your cancer recurs, it is normal to experience emotions such as disbelief or fear. If you are having these or other feelings of distress, it is important to talk about your emotions with your family and friends and health care team, and seek appropriate supportive services to help address the emotions that often come with a cancer diagnosis and its treatment.

Immunotherapy as a Treatment for Metastatic Bladder Cancer

Immunotherapy is a rapidly evolving approach to treating metastatic bladder cancer. This approach to treatment harnesses the patient's own immune system to fight cancer cells.

In May 2016 and February 2017, the U.S. Federal Drug Administration (FDA) approved the first two immunotherapy drugs for use in patients with metastatic bladder cancer. Many other immunotherapy drugs for use in patients with metastatic bladder cancer are currently under investigation — and it is likely that these drugs will play an increasingly larger role in treating metastatic bladder cancer in the near future. If you have been diagnosed with metastatic bladder cancer, you should discuss these emerging therapies with your medical oncologist.

The new immunotherapy drugs harness the patient's own immune system to fight cancer cells systemically (throughout the body). The ability of these drugs to attack cancer cells systemically is in contrast to another type of immunotherapy, called BCG, which is used to treat non-muscle-invasive bladder cancer. Unlike systemic immunotherapy, BCG is instilled directly into the bladder — and harnesses the immune system to fight cancer cells only in the bladder. (For a discussion of BCG, see chapter 6.)

Are Clinical Trials an Option for Metastatic Bladder Cancer?

Clinical trials may be an option for patients with metastatic bladder cancer. Taking part in a clinical trial gives patients access to new drugs and regimens before they are widely available. For these patients, clinical trials may offer hope for a better outcome.

When exploring your treatment options, ask your doctor if participating in a clinical trial is a treatment option.

WHAT ARE CLINICAL TRIALS?

To make scientific advances in treating bladder cancer, investigators conduct **clinical trials** — research studies that involve people and test new ways to prevent, detect, and treat bladder cancer. Clinical trials are used to determine the safety and effectiveness of new treatments and whether they are more effective than standard treatments. *Standard treatments* (also called *standards of care* or *best practices*) are treatments that experts agree are appropriate, accepted, and widely used.

Treatments studied in bladder cancer clinical trials include new immunotherapy medicines, new chemotherapy drugs, new combinations of existing drugs, different doses of currently used drugs, and new methods of treatment. There are also clinical trials that study new ways to reduce symptoms and manage treatment-related side effects.

Clinical trials are usually conducted in a series of steps, called *phases:*

- **Phase I** trials are conducted mainly to evaluate the safety of drugs and other interventions. They help determine the maximum dose that can be given safely, how the new treatment should be given, and whether the new treatment causes harmful side effects. Phase I trials usually enroll small groups of people (20 to 80) with advanced cancer who cannot be treated effectively with standard treatments, or for whom no standard treatment exists.

- **Phase II** trials test the effectiveness of a treatment and continue to evaluate its safety. These studies usually enroll a larger group of people (several hundred).

- **Phase III** trials compare the effectiveness and side effects of a new treatment with that of the standard treatment. If the results of a phase III trial show that the new treatment is more effective than the standard treatment and/or is easier to tolerate, it may become the new standard of care. Phase III trials usually involve large numbers of people (several hundred to several thousand). Participants are randomly assigned to either a control group (receive the standard treatment) or an investigational group (receive the treatment being studied). This type of trial is called a *controlled, randomized trial*.

To join a clinical trial, you must give *informed consent*. Each clinical trial has a written protocol (treatment plan), which describes in detail what will be done during the trial and the potential side effects. Be sure to carefully review the protocol before signing the informed consent form. Patients who participate in a clinical trial may stop participating at any time for personal or medical reasons.

For more information about clinical trials, see appendix C, "Bladder Cancer Resources."

When Is Radiation Therapy Used?

Radiation therapy appears to have minimal curative potential for patients with metastatic bladder cancer. However, radiation therapy may be used to relieve advanced bladder cancer symptoms, such as pain, in order to improve a patient's quality of life. This is called *palliative* radiation therapy. In addition, radiation may be used to treat patients with distant metastasis in a specific area, such as the bone.

What Is Palliative Care?

An integral part of bladder cancer care is *palliative care*, also called *supportive care* or *symptom management*, which addresses the physical, emotional, social, and spiritual needs of cancer patients and their families. Palliative care focuses on the treatment of pain and other symptoms, such as fatigue, nausea, loss of appetite, depression, and difficulty sleeping. The goal of palliative care is to improve the quality of life of patients and their families as they deal with a life-threatening disease. Palliative care utilizes a multidisciplinary approach to patient care, which may involve a palliative care doctor, palliative care nurse, social worker, registered dietician, chaplain, pharmacist, psychologist, and other health care professionals.

PART 5 SURVIVORSHIP

Part 5 consists of **Chapter 14**, which discusses the challenges patients face when making the transition from active treatment to follow-up care — and strategies for confronting these challenges.

CHAPTER 14

Bladder Cancer Survivorship

This chapter discusses the potential challenges and risks that face bladder cancer survivors as they transition from active treatment to post-treatment care, often called *survivorship* care. Included in this chapter is information and tools that you and your family can use to partner with your doctor to manage your long-term, post-treatment follow-up care and surveillance. There are also tips for taking a proactive role in your survivorship care to maximize your health and quality of life.

The term *cancer survivor* means different things to different people. For many people, a person is considered a cancer survivor from the time of cancer diagnosis through the balance of his or her life. For others, a cancer survivor is anyone who has been cancer-free for 5 or more years. And for others, a cancer survivor is anyone who has completed active treatment and has no evidence of disease. For purposes of this chapter, we define a bladder cancer survivor as anyone who has completed active treatment and has no evidence of disease.

When Active Treatment Ends — New Questions and Concerns

During active treatment, you will be focused on completing your therapy and managing any side effects — with the goal of curing your disease. Often this is a challenging time, particularly if you are undergoing complex treatments, such as a radical cystectomy or systemic chemotherapy. While undergoing treatment, you are likely to form close connections with your doctor and other members of your medical team. Your doctors and nurses will be close at hand to answer your questions and monitor your side effects. However, when treatment is over, you may feel that you have lost this strong connection to your medical team and sense a loss of control.

After successful treatment, you may have mixed emotions, ranging from relief that you no longer have evidence of active disease — to fear of the cancer returning. You may have questions about how quickly you can return to your normal activities and doubts about your ability to regain your former quality of life. Many survivors need time after treatment to think about the experience they have been through, how it has changed their lives, and what it means for their future.

Having survived bladder cancer often motivates people to re-examine their priorities and set new goals, such as spending more time with family and friends, changing careers, or adopting a healthier lifestyle. Each cancer survivor is unique and has his or her own style of coping with adversity. Many cancer survivors discover a deep reservoir of strength within themselves and their loved ones and feel a profound sense of gratitude for a second chance at life.

Bladder cancer survivors often face difficult challenges after treatment, even when there is no evidence of active disease. Because bladder cancer has a very high rate of recurrence, the fear of the disease returning is an ongoing concern for most bladder cancer survivors. Furthermore, the long-term or late side effects associated with complex treatments can take a heavy toll on patients and their families. As a proactive cancer survivor, you need to understand the potential risks and adverse effects associated with your bladder cancer diagnosis and its treatment, so you will be better prepared to manage your long-term, post-treatment health needs.

Questions to Ask When Active Treatment Ends

For many, the transition from active treatment to post-treatment care raises new questions and concerns. To prepare for this transition, you should ask your doctor the following questions:

- Who will be responsible for coordinating and monitoring my follow-up cancer care?

- What physical symptoms and side effects could I experience as a result of my cancer or its treatment?
- How likely is my cancer to recur and/or progress?
- What tests will be needed to monitor for recurrence of my disease, and how often will I need these tests?
- What is the recommended schedule for follow-up visits?
- What can I do to promote my health and well-being?
- Am I at risk for developing other primary cancers as a result of my cancer diagnosis and/or its treatment? If so, what can I do to prevent or screen for these cancers?
- What support services and resources are available during survivorship care?

Asking these questions, and asking them again until you understand the answers, is key to your post-treatment, survivorship care.

Remember, the goals of survivorship care are to maximize the longevity and quality of life of cancer survivors, and to address the unique physical, emotional, and social needs associated with a cancer diagnosis and its treatment.

Understanding Your Ongoing Cancer Risks

An essential part of follow-up care is surveillance for disease recurrence and/or progression, and monitoring for second cancers. As a bladder cancer survivor, you are at risk for a recurrence of your primary cancer; the development of cancer in another part of your urinary tract; and, rarely, the development of a second cancer (a new primary cancer) related to certain cancer treatments.

Bladder Cancer Recurrence and/or Progression

Recurrence refers to a return of cancer after a period in which there is no detectable disease. If when the cancer returns (recurs), it is a higher stage (more extensive) and/or a higher grade (more aggressive) than the original cancer, then it is said to have *progressed*.

Because recurrence of bladder cancer is common, all survivors require lifelong monitoring, usually by the doctor who provided their treatment. Since all bladder cancer survivors are at risk of cancer recurrence and/or progression, surveillance will be a key part of your lifelong, follow-up care.

Your individual risks of recurrence and/or progression will depend on your initial diagnosis and response to treatment. Based on your level of risk, your doctor will recommend a schedule of follow-up visits and surveillance tests and procedures to monitor for recurrent disease. It will be important for you to schedule follow-up visits and tests in a timely fashion, since early detection usually leads to better outcomes.

Cancer in Another Part of Your Urinary System

Bladder cancer that originates in the urothelial cells of the bladder lining is called *urothelial* bladder cancer. Urothelial cells line other parts of the urinary system as well — the kidneys, ureters, and urethra. When urothelial cancer develops in one part of the urinary system, such as the bladder, there is a risk of it developing in another part of the urinary system, as well. Therefore, once you have been diagnosed with urothelial cancer of the bladder, you will need to be monitored for urothelial cancer in other parts of your urinary system, as well.

Second Cancers

A *second cancer* refers to the development of a different type of primary cancer. Some treatments for bladder cancer, such as certain chemotherapy drugs, are associated with an increased risk of developing a second cancer. If you have received a treatment that is associated with the development of a second cancer, or if you have a genetic predisposition to a particular type of cancer, your doctor will recommend screening, as appropriate, to monitor for the disease.

Creating a Survivorship Care Plan

The landmark report *From Cancer Patient to Cancer Survivor: Lost in Transition* was released in 2005 by the Institute of Medicine (IOM) and National Research Council of the National Academies and published in 2006 by the National Academies Press. The book raises awareness of the adverse consequences of cancer and its treatment and identifies strategies for achieving the best possible outcomes for cancer survivors. It focuses on the physical, psychological, and social needs of cancer patients as they transition from primary treatment to post-treatment, survivorship care. You can read the report online or get a free PDF download of the book at *http://www.nationalacademies.org/hmd/Reports/2005/From-Cancer-Patient-to-Cancer-Survivor-Lost-in-Transition.aspx.*

From Cancer Patient to Cancer Survivor: Lost in Transition includes a recommendation that doctors provide cancer survivors, upon completion of primary treatment, with a ***survivorship care plan*** made up of two parts: a record of care and a follow-up care plan. A survivorship care plan is a tool for organizing the components of post-treatment care and making a plan for providing this care. Ideally, your survivorship care plan will facilitate and guide all aspects of your long-term, follow-up care, and answer any questions you have about your ongoing care.

The information that should be included in a survivorship care plan's *record of care* and *follow-up care plan* for bladder cancer survivors (discussed below) will vary according to the individual situation.

Record of Care

After cancer treatment, you should ask your doctor for a comprehensive, written summary of your bladder cancer diagnosis and treatment, including the following:

- Date of your diagnosis.
- Detailed records of all diagnostic tests and the results of these tests, including copies of all surgical, imaging, pathology, and urine cytology reports.
- Detailed information about your diagnosis, including the cell type(s), stage and grade, and number, size, and location of tumors.
- Detailed records of all your treatments, including surgical procedures, intravesical drug therapy, systemic chemotherapy, and radiation therapy. These records should include the dates and descriptions of all treatments — including agents used, treatment regimens, dosages, response to treatment, and related side effects or complications. If you participated in a clinical trial, your records should include the identifying number and title of the clinical trial.
- Record of all supportive services provided, including psychological, social, and nutritional services.

- Names and contact information of all health care providers and facilities involved in your care, including providers of psychological, social, nutritional, and other health services.
- Name and contact information of the doctor who is responsible for coordinating your bladder cancer care.

Follow-up Care Plan

Your specific health risks and needs after treatment will be determined by the stage of your disease at diagnosis, the treatments you received, your response to those treatments, and your overall health. The higher your stage at diagnosis, and the more complex the treatments you received, the more complex your follow-up care needs are likely to be.

To help plan for your individualized survivorship care, the following should be included in your follow-up care plan (will vary according to your individual situation):

- Name and contact information of the doctor who will be responsible for coordinating and monitoring your follow-up bladder cancer care.
- Schedule of follow-up visits recommended by your doctor (usually these will occur at regular intervals, such as every 3 months, every 6 months, or once a year).
- Schedule of procedures and tests recommended to monitor for cancer recurrence and second cancers.
- Symptoms you should watch for in connection with cancer recurrence and second cancers.
- Potential long-term and late side effects associated with your cancer and its treatment — such as urinary tract infection, blood clots, lymphedema, incontinence, change in sexual function, change in bowel habits, and fatigue — and symptoms to watch for in connection with these conditions.
- For patients with an ileal conduit reconstruction, a schedule of follow-up visits with an ET (enterostomal therapy) nurse.

- Specific recommendations for healthy behaviors, such as smoking cessation, diet, exercise, and weight management.
- Referrals to specific health care providers, if needed, such as a physical therapist to help with regaining continence after bladder removal; mental health professionals to assess and/or treat psychological or emotional symptoms; nutritional counseling; and/or oncology social workers to assist with social, employment, disability, insurance, or financial challenges.
- A list of cancer-related resources that provide information and/or support about survivorship issues.

Your follow-up care plan will need to clearly define the roles and responsibilities of the various specialists and primary care providers involved in your care, and specify who among them will carry out the various aspects of your follow-up care. Your plan should identify the doctor who will be responsible for coordinating your ongoing cancer care, preferably the doctor who treated your cancer.

It may be helpful to involve a trusted friend or family member in learning about your follow-up care needs, and to encourage him or her to advocate on your behalf (for example, to help you schedule appointments and tests when they are due). By asking for the help of a family member or friend, you will be adding a valuable member to your health care team. By actively participating in your own care, and encouraging others to support you on your journey, you will maximize the success of your survivorship care.

Tips for Taking a Proactive Role in Your Follow-up Care

In chapter 2, we discussed how to be a proactive patient so that you understand your diagnosis, make informed treatment decisions, and choose health care providers in whom you have confidence and trust to ensure that you get the best possible treatment outcomes. When treatment ends, you will need to build on that knowledge to maximize your health and quality of life. The following are some tips for taking a proactive role in your follow-up care.

- Take ownership of your follow-up care. Find the strategies that work for you to communicate with your doctors and nurses and other members of your health care team. Take advantage of

Internet-based resources that provide information about survivor-ship issues (see appendix C, "Bladder Cancer Resources"). Good information, together with effective communication skills, is what will enable you to take control of your follow-up care in a complex and often fragmented health care environment.

- Partner with your doctor by keeping a close eye on your health. Be sure to let your doctor know about any new symptoms, side effects, or other changes in your physical or emotional health. Do not wait for your doctor to ask before sharing this information. Keep a writ-ten record of when symptoms occur, how often they occur, and how long they last. Always let your doctor or nurse know about any new or changing symptoms, since they can be signs of potentially serious conditions, such as blood clots or infection, which require prompt medical attention.

- Be vigilant! The recurrent nature of bladder cancer means that you cannot let your guard down, no matter how well you feel or how busy you are. Be sure to schedule your follow-up visits and surveil-lance tests and procedures at intervals recommended by your doctor (every 3 months, every 6 months, once a year, and so on). Make sure you know what tests you will need to schedule, and be sure that the tests are scheduled far enough in advance so that the results will be available when you meet with your doctor. Do not wait to be con-tacted by your doctor's office to schedule your next follow-up visit. Instead, initiate the call yourself, or better still, schedule your next follow-up appointment and tests at the conclusion of your current appointment before you leave your doctor's office. Bring your calen-dar with you to facilitate scheduling.

- Consider joining a support group. Many people coping with illness find emotional and psychological support by connecting with oth-ers in similar situations. A support group consists of people with a similar disease who support each other by sharing information and experiences. There are many ways to connect with other bladder cancer survivors, either online or in person, either in a group setting or one-on-one (see appendix C, "Bladder Cancer Resources").

- Keep updated records of all of your follow-up care, and make revi-sions to your survivorship care plan, as needed. You will need to update the information, recommendations, and medical records that are included in your survivorship care plan to ensure that you and your health care providers have the most current information. Use your survivorship care plan as a way to track your progress in monitoring your health and meeting your health goals. By keeping abreast of your changing health needs and the steps you are taking to maximize your outcomes, you will feel more in control of your health and your life. This can be an effective way to cope with the anxiety and uncertainty associated with the fear of recurrence.

• Share your complete medical records with your various health care providers, including information about your cancer diagnosis, treatment history, and follow-up care. Although these records may seem unrelated, the information about your cancer and its treatment often has an impact on other aspects of your medical care.

PART 6   APPENDIXES

A. Bladder Cancer Risk Factors

B. Bladder Cancer Health Care Professionals

C. Bladder Cancer Resources

D. Glossary of Bladder Cancer Terms

Bladder Cancer Risk Factors

A risk factor for bladder cancer is anything that increases the likelihood of developing bladder cancer. Some risk factors, such as smoking and exposure to workplace chemicals, are controllable and can be changed. Other risk factors, such as age and gender, are not controllable and cannot be altered. Having a risk factor(s) for bladder cancer does not mean a person will develop the disease. However, it does mean that a person with a risk factor has a greater chance of developing bladder cancer than a person without a risk factor. Many people with risk factors never develop bladder cancer, while others with bladder cancer have no risk factors.

Smoking: Cigarette smoking is the greatest risk factor for bladder cancer and accounts for approximately 50% of bladder cancer in the United States. A strong link exists between the amount and duration of smoking. Smoking cigars and pipes also increases the risk of bladder cancer. Smokers are 2 to 3 times more likely to develop bladder cancer than nonsmokers.

Exposure to workplace chemicals: Workplace environments and occupations that expose workers to certain industrial chemicals increase the risk of bladder cancer. Workplace environments that increase the risk of bladder cancer include the dye, chemical, textile, leather, rubber, metal, paint, print, and dry cleaning industries. Occupations that increase the risk of bladder cancer include painters, printers, machinists, truck drivers (due to exposure to diesel fumes), and hairdressers (due to exposure to hair dyes). Good workplace safety practices can reduce these risks. It is estimated that 5%–10% of bladder cancer in the United States is caused by occupational exposure.

Age: The risk of bladder cancer increases with age. The average age of a person diagnosed with bladder cancer is 73, and 90% of people are diagnosed after age 55.

Gender: Men are approximately 3 times more likely to develop bladder cancer than women.

Race: Caucasians are approximately twice as likely to develop bladder cancer than African Americans or Hispanics. Asian Americans and American Indians have the lowest rates of bladder cancer.

Personal history of bladder cancer: People who have had bladder cancer have an increased risk of developing the disease again.

Chronic bladder problems: Bladder cancer is linked to long-term bladder irritation and inflammation caused by chronic bladder infections and bladder or kidney stones.

Arsenic exposure: Arsenic in drinking water has been linked to an increased risk of developing bladder cancer.

Previous cancer treatments: People treated with the chemotherapy drug Cytoxan (cyclophasphamide) have a higher risk of developing bladder cancer. People who have been treated with radiation to the pelvis for a previous cancer may have an elevated risk of developing bladder cancer.

Parasitic infection: Infection with certain parasites (particularly schistosomiasis) found in untreated drinking water in tropical regions of the world (not in the United States) increases the risk of bladder cancer.

Family history: It is rare for bladder cancer to run in families.

Diet: There is no clear evidence that dietary factors increase the risk of developing bladder cancer.

Bladder Cancer Health Care Professionals

Caring for patients with bladder cancer draws on the skills, expertise, and talents of health care professionals from many disciplines. It is important to choose medical specialists who have experience and expertise in treating bladder cancer. The following is a list of the different types of health care professionals and the roles they play in treating patients with bladder cancer.

Primary care doctor: A doctor, such as a family practitioner or internist, who treats a wide variety of medical conditions. During a routine physical examination, your primary care doctor may detect a symptom(s) associated with bladder cancer. If the symptom is not caused by a urinary tract infection or other benign condition, your primary care doctor should refer you to a urologist to determine whether or not you have bladder cancer.

Urologist: A doctor who specializes in treating diseases of the male and female urinary tract and male reproductive organs. Urologists have completed residency training in general urology.

Urologic oncologist: Urologic oncology is a branch of medicine that specializes in the diagnosis and treatment of urologic cancers, such as bladder cancer. A urologic oncologist is a urologist with advanced surgical training and medical education in urologic cancers. Urologic oncologists are surgical oncologists. They specialize in the diagnosis and treatment of cancers of the male and female urinary tract, including bladder cancer, and cancers of the male reproductive organs. Bladder removal surgery, called radical cystectomy, is the gold standard treatment for patients with muscle-invasive bladder cancer. It is a complex surgery requiring the skills of a urologic oncologist who performs a high volume of these operations. In most cases, a urologic oncologist will manage the patient's care, and make referrals, as needed, to other health care professionals, such as a medical oncologist and/or a radiation oncologist.

Medical oncologist: A physician who specializes in the treatment of cancer with systemic chemotherapy and other cancer-killing drugs. If you are undergoing systemic chemotherapy, you will be under the care of a medical oncologist, who will recommend a chemotherapy regimen and monitor your response to treatment and any adverse side affects.

Radiation oncologist: A doctor who specializes in the treatment of cancer using radiation therapy. Radiation therapy is given concurrently with systemic chemotherapy (called chemoradiation) during bladder preservation therapy.

Radiologist: A doctor who specializes in the use of imaging technologies, such as CT (computed tomography) and MRI (magnetic resonance imaging), to evaluate areas inside the body. When you undergo imaging tests, such as a CT scan or an MRI, a radiologist will interpret the scans to determine if there is evidence of bladder cancer.

Pathologist: A doctor who specializes in identifying cancer by examining cells and tissues under a microscope. Surgically removed tissue samples (biopsies) are examined by a pathologist to determine if bladder cancer is present.

Cytopathologist: A doctor who specializes in analyzing cells found in body fluids, such as urine. A cytopathologist examines cells from a urine sample under a microscope to determine if any cells are cancerous. This is called *urine cytology.*

Enterostomal therapy (ET) nurse: An ET nurse, also called an *enterostomal therapist* or *ostomy nurse,* is trained to care for patients with stomas. If you have an ileal conduit, an ET nurse will teach you how to care for your stoma and change your ostomy bag.

Anesthesiologist: A doctor who specializes in giving drugs or other agents to prevent pain during a surgical procedure.

Oncology nurse: A nurse who specializes in the treatment and care of cancer patients. If you are having systemic chemotherapy, an oncology nurse will care for you.

Oncology social worker: A health professional who provides social and emotional support for cancer patients and their families. Oncology social workers make referrals to support services that address the social, psychological, employment, disability, insurance, and financial needs of cancer patients and their families.

Bladder Cancer Resources

The following are organizations and websites that offer educational materials, support, and advocacy for people diagnosed with bladder cancer and their families and friends.

Bladder Cancer Patient Advocacy, Education, and Support

www.bcan.org

The website for *BCAN*, which stands for *Bladder Cancer Advocacy Network*. BCAN was founded in 2005 by Diane Zipursky Quale and the late John Quale, who died in 2007 after a battle with bladder cancer. BCAN is the only national advocacy organization for those impacted by bladder cancer. Its mission is to educate and support bladder cancer patients and their families, advance bladder cancer research, and raise public awareness of the disease. BCAN wants to make sure that no one who is diagnosed with bladder cancer feels alone in dealing with his or her disease. You can go to the BCAN website or call the toll-free number, 888-901-BCAN (2226).

http://www.bcan.org/learn/online-resource-library

BCAN's *Online Resource Library*, with links to free educational webinars and videos; the BCAN Connection, an information and referral phone line for bladder cancer patients and their loved ones, staffed by BCAN volunteers; BCAN Survivor2Survivor, a program that connects patients newly diagnosed with bladder cancer with patient volunteers who have faced a similar diagnosis and treatment options; and Inspire, an online bladder cancer support group and discussion community for bladder cancer patients and their loved ones.

www.inspire.com/groups/bladder-cancer-advocacy-network

Inspire is BCAN's online bladder cancer support group and discussion community hosted by Inspire. More than 20,000 patients and their loved ones are members of this online community. Members can connect with others impacted by bladder cancer to ask questions, share information and resources, and offer support and encouragement.

Other Cancer-Related Organizations and Websites

www.cancer.net

The *American Society of Clinical Oncology's (ASCO)'s* patient information website, aimed at helping patients and families make informed health care decisions. To find information about bladder cancer on this website, click on "Types of Cancer" and then click on "Bladder Cancer." The web page is *www .cancer.net/cancer-types/bladder-cancer.*

www.cancer.gov

The website of the *National Cancer Institute (NCI)* — the federal government's principal agency for cancer research and training. The NCI is part of the National Institutes of Health, the world's premier medical research organization. The NCI collects and disseminates information on cancer detection, diagnosis, treatment, prevention, and survivorship. It supports a national network of cancer centers, called the NCI-designated cancer centers, serving cancer patients throughout the U.S. For information about bladder cancer, click on "Cancer Types," and then under "Common Cancer Types," click on "Bladder Cancer." The web page is *www.cancer.gov/types/bladder.*

http://cancercenters.cancer.gov/center/cancercenters

Use this link to search for an *NCI-designated cancer center* in your area. NCI-designated cancer centers deliver cutting-edge cancer treatments in communities throughout the United States. There are 69 NCI-designated cancer centers in 35 states and the District of Columbia. Each year, more than 250,000 cancer patients are treated at NCI-designated cancer centers and thousands of cancer patients are enrolled in cancer clinical trials at these centers.

www.cancer.org

The website of the *American Cancer Society* (ACS), a nationwide health organization dedicated to helping people who face cancer. The ACS supports research, patient services, early detection, treatment, and education. To find information about bladder cancer, click on "Learn About Cancer." Then, under "Select a Cancer Type," choose "Bladder Cancer." The web page for bladder cancer is *www.cancer.org/cancer/bladdercancer/index.*

www.nccn.org

The website of the *National Comprehensive Cancer Network* (NCCN), an alliance of 26 leading cancer centers in the United States. Its mission is to improve the quality, effectiveness, and efficiency of care provided to cancer patients.

Information About Clinical Trials

www.clinicaltrials.gov

A database for publicly and privately supported clinical trials on cancer and other diseases conducted in the U.S. and throughout the world. The website lists NCI-supported cancer trials as well as cancer trials sponsored by pharmaceutical and biotech companies.

http://www.cancer.gov/about-cancer/treatment/clinical-trials

A web page on the National Cancer Institute (NCI) website, providing information for patients and caregivers about participating in clinical trials.

http://www.cancer.gov/clinicaltrials/search

Use this link to search for *NCI-supported clinical trials.* NCI-supported clinical trials are cancer trials sponsored or otherwise financially supported by the National Cancer Institute (NCI).

Support for Cancer Patients and Their Families

www.cancercare.org

CancerCare is a leading national organization that provides professional support services to help cancer patients and survivors cope with the emotional and practical challenges facing cancer patients and their families. CancerCare offers free, professional support services, including counseling, support groups, educational workshops, and financial assistance.

www.cancersupportcommunity.org

Cancer Support Community provides free, professional programs of emotional support, education, and hope for people impacted by cancer. The Cancer Support Community Affiliate Network consists of 44 licensed affiliates at 170 locations. To find an affiliate at a location closest to you, click on "Find an Affiliate."

www.cancerhopenetwork.org

The *Cancer Hope Network* matches its more than 400 Support Volunteers with cancer patients and cancer caregivers who face similar challenges related to a cancer diagnosis. Matches are made based on factors such as diagnosis and treatment plan, giving patients and caregivers an opportunity to speak with Support Volunteers whose experience is similar to their own.

Online Cancer Support and Discussion Communities

www.inspire.com/groups/bladder-cancer-advocacy-network

Inspire is BCAN's online bladder cancer support group and discussion community for patients and their loved ones. Members of this online community connect with others impacted by bladder cancer to ask questions, share information and resources, and offer support and encouragement.

www.cancer.org/treatment/supportprogramsservices
/onlinecommunities

A web page on the American Cancer Society's website with links to online communities and support, including the *Cancer Survivors Network* and *I Can Cope®*.

www.cancersupportcommunity.org/online-support

The Living Room is the Cancer Support Community's online support community, where anyone impacted by cancer can find support, education, and hope.

https://www.facebook.com/bladdercancersupportgroup

The link to the *Bladder Cancer Support Group* on Facebook.

www.acor.org

This is the website for *ACOR*, which stands for *Association of Cancer Online Resources*. ACOR's 142 online cancer communities provide a forum for patients, caregivers, family members, and friends to share information and support pertaining to specific types of cancer. Bladder Cancer Cafe is ACOR's bladder cancer discussion community for people diagnosed with bladder cancer, their family members, and friends. The link to Bladder Cancer Cafe is *www.acor .org/listservs/join/13*.

Support for Patients with Stomas

www.ostomy.org

The website of the *United Ostomy Association of America, Inc.* (UOAA), an association of more than 340 UOAA-affiliated support groups dedicated to improving the quality of life for people with an ostomy. The UOAA provides information, advocacy, and support for patients and their loved ones who have had or are going to have ostomy or related surgeries. To find the UOAA-affiliated support group nearest to you, click on "Support Groups."

Cancer Survivorship

http://www.nationalacademies.org/hmd/Reports/2005/From-Cancer -Patient-to-Cancer-Survivor-Lost-in-Transition.aspx

Use this link to download a free copy of *From Cancer Patient to Cancer Survivor: Lost in Transition*. This report was released in 2005 by the Institute of Medicine and the National Research Council of the National Academies of Sciences, Engineering, and Medicine (the Academies) and published in 2006 by the National Academies Press. The book raises awareness of the adverse consequences of cancer and its treatment and identifies strategies to achieve the best possible outcomes for cancer survivors. The Institute of Medicine (IOM) was established in 1970 and was renamed the National Academy of Medicine in 2015.

www.canceradvocacy.org

The website for the *National Coalition for Cancer Survivorship* (NCCS), which advocates for the millions of Americans who share the experience of cancer survivorship — living with, through, and beyond a cancer diagnosis. Click on "Resources" to find information on a range of topics of interest to cancer survivors, including "Talking with Your Doctor," "Advocating for Yourself," "Employment Rights," and "Health Insurance."

Urologic Health

www.urologyhealth.org

The website of the *Urology Care Foundation* — the official foundation of the American Urological Association (formerly the American Urological Association Foundation). The mission of the Urology Care Foundation is to advance urologic research and education. It strives to provide up-to-date, accurate urologic health information to patients and the public. To find information on bladder cancer, click on "Educational Materials," then click on "Search for Patient Materials." Then scroll down to "Bladder Cancer Patient Guide" for a free copy of a 12-page guide called *Non-Muscle-Invasive Bladder Cancer: A Patient Guide.*

Health and Medical Information Databases

http://www.nlm.nih.gov

The website for the *U.S. National Library of Medicine* (NLM), the world's largest medical library, including millions of books and journals on all aspects of medicine and health care. The NLM offers free, web-based services to the public, including MEDLINE/PubMed, PubMed Health, and ClinicalTrials.gov.

http://pubmed.gov

MEDLINE/PubMed is a free database managed by the National Library of Medicine. You can search this database for free *abstracts* — short technical summaries — of more than 25 million scientific articles about medicine and health from biomedical journals.

www.ncbi.nim.gov/pubmedhealth

PubMed Health is a service of the National Center for Biotechnology Information (NCBI) of the U.S. National Library of Medicine (NLM). This is a public service providing information for consumers and clinicians on the prevention and treatment of disease. Includes summaries and full-text reports on clinical effectiveness research (research on what works).

Website for This Book

bladdercancerbook.org

The website for *Bladder Cancer: A Patient-Friendly Guide to Understanding Your Diagnosis and Treatment Options* by David Pulver, Mark Schoenberg, MD, and Fran Pulver.

Note to the Reader

The resources listed in this appendix are meant for informational purposes only and do not constitute an endorsement of any websites, web pages, or other sources. Please note that the URLs for websites and web pages in this appendix are subject to change. The authors and publisher have no control over and assume no responsibility for third-party websites or web pages or their content.

Glossary of Bladder Cancer Terms

A

Adenocarcinoma: A rare type of bladder cancer, which accounts for about 2% of bladder cancer diagnosed in the United States.

Adjuvant chemotherapy: Chemotherapy given after primary treatment (for example, systemic chemotherapy given after a radical cystectomy) to reduce the risk of recurrence of the disease.

Artificial urinary sphincter (AUS): A medical device that can be surgically implanted in men and women with a neobladder who fail to regain continence after a radical cystectomy.

Atypical cells: When cells from a urine sample are examined under a microscope during urine cytology, the finding can be malignant (cancerous), benign (noncancerous), or atypical. A finding of *atypical* means the cells are neither cancerous nor benign. The significance of atypical cells is often unclear. Such a finding may prompt the doctor to order additional diagnostic tests and/or repeat the urine cytology.

B

BCG: Stands for *bacillus Calmette-Guérin*. BCG is a type of intravesical immunotherapy, which uses the body's own immune system to kill bladder cancer cells. It is a primary treatment for CIS. *See also* **Intravesical drug therapy**

Benign: Cells are noncancerous, meaning there are no cancer cells.

Biopsy: A sample of cells or tissues removed from the body for examination under a microscope by a pathologist, a doctor trained to identify cancer and other diseases by examining cells and tissues under a microscope. Also called *specimen. See also* **Random biopsies**

Bladder: A hollow, balloon-shaped organ located behind the pelvic bones, surrounded by several organs. The bladder stores urine, the liquid waste produced by the kidneys. As a storehouse for urine, the bladder is constantly filling up and emptying. *See chapter 3, figures 3.6 (male) and 3.7 (female).*

Bladder lining: The innermost layer of the bladder wall. Bladder cancer originates in the bladder lining. Also called *urothelium, mucosa,* and *transitional epithelium. See chapter 3, figure 3.8 and chapter 5, figure 5.1.*

Bladder cancer: Cancer that begins in the bladder lining (urothelium).

Bladder preservation therapy: An alternative to a radical cystectomy in carefully selected patients. Bladder preservation therapy treats bladder cancer without removing the bladder. Also called *bladder-sparing therapy* or *trimodality therapy (TMT).*

Bladder-sparing therapy. *See* **Bladder preservation therapy**

Bladder wall: The bladder has a thick wall composed of several layers, called the *bladder wall.* The innermost layer is the *bladder lining,* also called the *urothelium, mucosa,* and *transitional epithelium.* Next to the bladder lining is the *lamina propria,* also called *submucosa.* Outside the lamina propria is the *muscle,* also called *muscularis propria.* Around the muscle is the *fat,* also called *perivesical fat. See chapter 3, figure 3.8.*

Bladder washing: A method of obtaining a urine sample by draining urine from the bladder.

Blue light cystoscopy: A relatively new procedure increasingly being used to better diagnose patients with suspected or known non-muscle-invasive bladder cancer. A blue light cystoscopy uses an imaging solution and blue light (in addition to white light) to improve the visibility of tumors. Also called *fluorescence cystoscopy.*

Bowel. *See* **Intestine**

C

Cancer: Cancer is characterized by uncontrolled growth of abnormal cells, which form tumors. Also called *carcinoma*.

Carcinoma. *See* **Cancer**

Carcinoma in situ (CIS): Flat, high-grade tumors confined to the bladder lining (urothelium). CIS has the potential to spread to other parts of the body rapidly and unpredictably. Also called *TIS* (tumor in situ).

Catheter: A thin, flexible tube used to instill (introduce) or drain (withdraw) fluids. *See also* **Catheterize**

Catheterize: To use a catheter to instill or drain fluids. *See also* **Catheter**

Centimeter: Tumors are measured in centimeters, abbreviated *cm*. A centimeter is a unit of length in the metric system. There are 2 ½ centimeters in one inch.

Chemoradiation: Use of systemic chemotherapy and radiation therapy concurrently (at the same time) to kill cancer cells.

Chemotherapy: The use of drugs to kill cancer cells.

CIS. *See* **Carcinoma in situ (CIS)**

Cisplatin: A systemic chemotherapy drug used to treat metastatic bladder cancer. *See also* **GC** and **MVAC**

Clinical stage: The doctor's best estimate of the extent of the cancer, based on what is learned from a physical examination, cystoscopy, TURBT, examination of biopsies under a microscope, and imaging tests.

Clinical trial: A research study that tests new ways to prevent, detect, or treat cancer and other diseases in people. Also called *clinical study*.

Continence: The ability to control the flow of urine to the outside of the body.

Continent catheterizable reservoir: One of three types of urinary tract reconstructions created during a radical cystectomy after the bladder is removed. During reconstruction, the surgeon makes a small opening (stoma) in the abdominal wall. Patients with a continent catheterizable reservoir empty urine from an internal reservoir (pouch) by inserting a catheter into the stoma. An *Indiana pouch* is a type of continent catheterizable reservoir. *See also chapter 10, figure 10.3.*

CT scan: A CT (computed tomography) scan uses a computer linked to an X-ray machine to create detailed images of internal organs, bones, soft tissue, and blood vessels.

CT urogram: A specialized CT scan, which provides more detailed images of the urinary tract than those created by a conventional CT scan.

Curative: A treatment given with the intention of curing the patient of the disease.

Cure: In bladder cancer, the term *cure* means there is no evidence of cancer for 5 years or longer. Achieving a cure does not mean the cancer will not come back (recur), but recurrence is much less likely in patients who are cancer-free for 5 or more years.

Cystoscope: A thin, tube-like instrument that is passed through the urethra to visually examine the lower urinary tract (bladder and urethra) during a cystoscopy. *See chapter 4, figure 4.1. See also* **Cystoscopy**

Cystoscopy: A procedure that uses an instrument called a *cystoscope* to visually examine the lower urinary tract (bladder and urethra). *See chapter 4, figure 4.1. See also* **Cystoscopy**

Cystectomy. *See* **Radical cystectomy**

Cytology. *See* **Urine cytology**

D

Distant metastasis: In bladder cancer, the spread of cancer from the bladder to a distant site, such as the liver, lung, bone, or distant lymph nodes.

Dome: The roof of the bladder. *See chapter 3, figures 3.6 (male) and 3.7 (female).*

E

ED. *See* **Erectile dysfunction**

Erectile dysfunction (ED): A condition that can occur in men as a result of the removal of the prostate during a radical cystectomy. ED is the inability to have or maintain an erection during sexual intercourse. Also called *impotence.*

F

Fat: The tissue around the muscle of the bladder wall. Also called *perivesical fat. See chapter 3, figure 3.8 and chapter 5, figure 5.1.*

First-line treatment: The initial treatment. Also called *primary* treatment.

Five-year survival rate: The percentage of patients who are alive 5 years after diagnosis of their disease.

Fluorescence cystoscopy. *See* **Blue light cystoscopy**

Focal: In bladder cancer, means the tumor is located in one area.

Foley catheter: A flexible tube (catheter) inserted through the urethra to drain urine from the bladder or neobladder. Also called *urethral catheter.*

G

Genes: Every cell contains thousands of genes, each of which has a set of instructions for making proteins. Many cancers are thought to arise from changes (mutations) in the DNA of genes that interfere with the orderly growth and division of cells.

GC: An acronym for gemcitabine and cisplatin — two chemotherapy drugs used in combination to treat metastatic bladder cancer.

Grade: The grade of bladder cancer indicates the aggressiveness of the disease. The grading system for bladder cancer is *low grade* and *high grade. See also* **High-grade bladder cancer** and **Low-grade bladder cancer**

H

Hematuria: A condition in which there is blood in the urine. Hematuria can be either *gross* (visible to the naked eye) or *microscopic* (visible only under a microscope). Hematuria is the most common symptom of bladder cancer.

High-grade bladder cancer: *High-grade* cancer cells appear highly abnormal when viewed under a microscope. High-grade bladder cancer has a high risk of invading the deeper layers of the bladder wall and spreading to other parts of the body. High-grade cancer cells are aggressive, with a high risk of recurrence and/or progression.

I

Ileal conduit: One of three types of urinary tract reconstructions created during a radical cystectomy after the bladder is removed. During reconstruction, the surgeon makes a small opening (stoma) in the abdominal wall through which urine exits the body. Patients with an ileal conduit wear an external pouch, called an *ostomy bag*, to collect the urine. The ostomy bag must be emptied several times a day. *See chapter 10, figure 10.1.*

Ileum: A portion of the small intestine. Surgeons use a section of the ileum to create a urinary tract reconstruction during a radical cystectomy.

Immunotherapy: Uses substances that stimulate the body's own immune system to fight cancer and other diseases.

Impotence. *See* **Erectile Dysfunction (ED)**

Incontinence: The inability to control the flow of urine to the outside of the body.

Indiana Pouch. *See* **Continent Catheterizable Reservoir**

Infusion. *See* **Intravenous (IV)**

Instillation: Introducing a liquid into a body cavity or passage, where it is allowed to remain for a period of time. Intravesical drugs, such as BCG, are instilled (introduced) into the bladder through a catheter inserted into the urethra.

Interferon: A type of immunotherapy that uses cytokines (proteins produced by white blood cells) to stimulate an immune response against cancer cells.

Intestine: A long, tube-like organ in the abdomen. Consists of two parts, the small intestine and large intestine. Also called *bowel.*

Intravenous (IV): A way of delivering a drug or substance into the bloodstream by inserting a small tube *into a vein.* Also called *infusion.*

Intravesical: Means *within* or *inside the bladder.*

Intravesical chemotherapy. *See* **Intravesical drug therapy**

Intravesical drug therapy: Medications instilled into the bladder through a catheter inserted into the urethra. Immunotherapy drugs, such as BCG, instilled into the bladder are called *intravesical immunotherapy.* Chemotherapy drugs, such as mytomycin C, instilled into the bladder are called *intravesical chemotherapy. See chapter 6, figure 6.2.*

Intravesical immunotherapy. *See* **Intravesical drug therapy**

K

Kidneys: A pair of bean-shaped organs located near the middle of the back, just below the rib cage. *See chapter 3, figure 3.5.*

L

Lamina propria: Connective tissue that separates the bladder lining (urothelium) from the muscle (muscularis propria). Also called *submucosa.* Cancer that invades the lamina propria is at high risk of invading the muscle. *See chapter 3, figure 3.8 and chapter 5, figure 5.1.*

Left lateral wall: The wall of the bladder, located on the left side of the trigone. *See chapter 3, figures 3.6 (male) and 3.7 (female).*

Lesion. *See* **Tumor**

Lower urinary tract: The bladder and urethra are in the lower urinary tract. *See chapter 3, figures 3.1 (male) and 3.3 (female).*

Low-grade bladder cancer: *Low-grade* cancer cells closely resemble normal cells when viewed under a microscope. Low-grade bladder cancer is usually not an aggressive cancer, with a low risk of progressing beyond the bladder lining (urothelium). However, it has a high risk of recurrence and must be closely monitored.

Lymph nodes: Small, bean-shaped structures, made of lymphatic tissue, scattered throughout the body, including the pelvis, abdomen, and chest. *See chapter 3, figure 3.9.*

Lymphatic system: Part of the body's immune system, which fights infection and disease. The lymphatic system is made up of lymph (excess fluid), lymphatic vessels, and lymph nodes.

Lymphatic vessels: A system of interconnecting channels that transports lymph (excess fluid) into the blood. Bladder cancer can spread from the bladder to other sites in the body through the lymphatic vessels.

M

MVAC: An acronym for methotrexate, vinblastine, doxorubicin (Adriamycin), and cisplatin — four systemic chemotherapy drugs used in combination to treat metastatic bladder cancer.

Malignant: Cells are cancerous, meaning that cancer is present in the cells.

Metastatic bladder cancer: Bladder cancer that has spread from the original (primary) site (the bladder) to nearby lymph nodes and/or distant sites in the body, such as the lung, liver, bone, or distant lymph nodes. *See also* **Micrometastatic bladder cancer**

Metastasize: When cancer cells metastasize, they spread from the original site (the bladder) to another part of the body through the lymphatic system.

Micrometastatic bladder cancer: Metastatic bladder cancer that is too small to be seen by the naked eye (microscopic). *See also* **Metastatic bladder cancer**

Micropapillary carcinoma: A rare and aggressive variant (version) of urothelial bladder cancer.

Millimeter: Small tumors are measured in millimeters, abbreviated *mm*. A millimeter is a unit of length in the metric system. There are 10 millimeters in 1 centimeter. There are 25 millimeters in one inch.

Mitomycin C: A type of intravesical chemotherapy. Mitomycin C is instilled into the bladder to treat non-muscle-invasive bladder cancer. *See also* **Intravesical drug theapy**

MRI: An MRI (magnetic resonance imaging) uses magnetic fields to create detailed pictures of areas inside the body.

Multifocal: In bladder cancer, means there are tumors in multiple areas of the bladder.

Mucosa. *See* **Bladder lining**

Muscle: The outermost layer of the bladder wall. Composed of thick, smooth, muscle bundles. Also called *muscularis propria. See chapter 3, figure 3.8 and chapter 5, figure 5.1.*

Muscle-invasive bladder cancer: Bladder cancer that invades the muscle (muscularis propria) of the bladder wall. Muscle-invasive bladder cancer also includes cancer that has extended past the muscle to the fat (perivesical fat) and/or adjacent organs, such as the prostate, vagina, or uterus. *See chapter 7, figure 7.1.*

Muscularis propria. *See* **Muscle**

Mutation: A change in the DNA sequence of genes. Many cancers are thought to arise from changes (mutations) in the DNA of genes that interfere with the orderly growth and division of cells.

N

Negative: When the results of a test is negative, it means that no cancer is detected.

Neoadjuvant chemotherapy: Systemic chemotherapy given prior to surgery.

Neobladder: One of three types of urinary tract reconstructions created during a radical cystectomy after the bladder is removed. During reconstruction, the surgeon creates an internal reservoir for storing urine inside the body. A neobladder is the only type of urinary tract reconstruction that allows the patient to empty urine through the urethra. Also called *orthotopic neobladder. See chapter 10, figure 10.2.*

Non-metastatic bladder cancer: There is no evidence that bladder cancer has metastasized (spread) to nearby lymph nodes and/or distant sites, such as the lung, liver, bone, or distant lymph nodes.

Non-muscle-invasive bladder cancer: Bladder cancer that is contained within the bladder lining (urothelium) or has grown through the bladder lining into the lamina propria (submucosa) — but has *not* invaded the muscle (muscularis propria). *See chapter 6, figure 6.1.*

O

Orthotopic neobladder. *See* **Neobladder**

Ostomy: A procedure that creates a surgical opening (hole) from the inside to the outside of the body. This opening is called a *stoma* or an *ostomy.*

Ostomy bag: An external pouch, called an *ostomy bag,* worn by patients with an ileal conduit to collect urine that drains from their stoma. An ostomy bag must be emptied several times a day and changed every 3 to 4 days.

P

Papillary tumors: Look like seaweed or coral attached by stems to the bladder lining (urothelium). These tumors grow toward the hollow center of the bladder, away from the deeper layers of the bladder wall.

Partial cystectomy: A surgical procedure to remove a portion of the bladder, leaving the functioning of the bladder intact. About 5% of patients with muscle-invasive bladder cancer are candidates for a partial cystectomy.

Pathologic stage: Based on a microscopic examination of the tissues and organs removed during a radical cystectomy, a pathologist can determine the *pathologic* stage of the cancer.

Pathology report: A pathologist writes a *pathology report,* indicating whether bladder cancer is present and, if so, the cell type, grade (low grade or high grade), and stage (depth and extent) of the disease. The pathology report is based on a microscopic examination of cells, tissues, and organs removed from the body.

Perivesical: Means *around the bladder.*

Perivesical fat. *See* **Fat**

PET scan: Stands for *positron emission tomography.* This is an imaging test that uses radioactive sugar to identify cancer cells. A small amount of radioactive sugar, called *tracer,* is injected into a vein at the beginning of the test. A scanner takes pictures of areas inside the body, which shows how cells absorb the sugar. Because cancer cells absorb more sugar than normal cells, cancer cells look different from normal cells.

PET-CT scan: An imaging test that combines the pictures from a PET (positron emission tomography) scan and a CT (computed tomography) scan to provide more detailed images of areas inside the body.

Positive: When the results of a test is positive, it means that cancer is present.

Posterior wall: The back wall of the bladder. *See chapter 3, figures 3.6 (male) and 3.7 (female).*

Primary site: The place in the body (such as the bladder) where the cancer originates.

Primary treatment. *See* **First-line treatment**

Proactive: As pertains to this book, *proactive* means an approach to getting health care in which health care consumers (you and your family) play an active role in your care. This includes educating yourself about your disease and treatment options, and participating in treatment decisions. It means anticipating problems, and taking actions to prevent or minimize them. The goal is to take control of your health care and get the best possible outcomes for your disease.

Prognosis: A forecast (prediction) of the likely outcome or course of a disease.

Progress: When talking about cancer, to *progress* means to get worse in terms of stage (growth or spread of the tumor) or grade (high grade vs. low grade).

Progression: A worsening of cancer to a higher stage or grade.

Protocol. *See* **Treatment plan**

R

Radiation therapy: The use of high-energy radiation to destroy cancer cells.

Radical cystectomy: A surgical procedure to remove the bladder. Also called a *cystectomy.* Other organs and tissues removed during a radical cystectomy include nearby lymph nodes and, in men, the prostate and seminal vesicles. The surgeon also reconstructs the lower urinary tract, called *urinary tract reconstruction,* to provide a way for urine to leave the body after the bladder is removed.

Random biopsies: The removal of random (normal looking) tissue samples (biopsies) for examination under a microscope. The purpose of taking random biopsies is to check for microscopic cancer, which is not visible to the naked eye. *See also* **Biopsy**

Recurrence: The return of cancer after a complete response (no evidence of disease).

Refractory disease: Cancer that does not respond to treatment (does not improve or gets worse). Also called *resistant disease.*

Regimen. *See* **Treatment plan**

Remission: The response to treatment is the disappearance of the tumor or a reduction in the amount of tumor. A complete response (also called *complete remission*) means there is no cancer detected in the body. A partial response (also called *partial remission*) means there is a decrease of more than 50% in the amount of cancer detected in the body.

Resect: To remove surgically.

Resectable: Can be removed surgically.

Resection: The surgical removal of tissues and organs.

Resectoscope: A thin, tube-like instrument equipped with special tools for taking biopsies and removing (resecting) tumors from the bladder wall. A resectoscope is used to perform a TURBT. *See chapter 4, figure 4.2. See also* **TURBT**

Residual cancer: Cancer that remains after treatment.

Resistant disease. *See* **Refractory disease**

Restaging TURBT: A TURBT that is repeated to re-evaluate the stage (depth and extent) of cancer in the lower urinary tract (bladder and urethra).

Response: An improvement as a result of treatment, such as a decrease in the size of the tumor.

Right lateral wall: The wall of the bladder located on the right side of the trigone. *See chapter 3, figures 3.6 and 3.7.*

Risk of recurrence: The likelihood of the tumor recurring (returning) after a complete response (no evidence of disease).

Risk of progression: The likelihood of the tumor progressing to a higher stage or grade.

S

Salvage radical cystectomy: A radical cystectomy (bladder removal surgery) that is performed after the primary (initial) treatment fails. For example, if bladder preservation therapy fails to eradicate the cancer, a salvage radical cystectomy may be considered.

Second opinion: A consultation with a different doctor to obtain another opinion. It is a common practice to get a second opinion about a cancer diagnosis and/or treatment options.

Second-line treatment: Treatment given after the primary (first-line) treatment fails to eradicate the disease.

Selection criteria: Factors that need be evaluated to determine if a patient is a suitable candidate for a treatment, such as a radical cystectomy or bladder preservation therapy.

Sensitivity: The sensitivity of a test for detecting cancer indicates the percentage of people with cancer who get positive test results. A test has a high rate of sensitivity when the test results are positive in a high percentage of patients with the disease. Another measure of a test is its *specificity. See* **Specificity**

Sessile tumors: Solid tumors. Sessile tumors have the ability to infiltrate (grow through) the bladder lining (urothelium) into the deeper layers of the bladder wall and spread to other parts of the body.

Side effect: A problem that occurs as a result of treatment. Side effects can be short-term (go away shortly after treatment), long-term (last for months or years after treatment ends), or late (occur months or years after treatment ends).

Specificity: The specificity of a test for detecting cancer indicates the percentage of people without cancer who get negative test results. A test has a high rate of specificity when the test results are negative in a high percentage of patients without the disease. Another measure of a test is its *sensitivity. See also* **Sensitivity**

Sphincter. *See* **Urinary sphincter**

Squamous cell carcinoma: This type of bladder cancer begins in the squamous cells and accounts for about 5% of bladder cancer in the United States.

Squamous cell carcinoma is more common in parts of the world (i.e., Africa) where a parasite, called a *schistosome*, is endemic.

Stable disease: There is neither an increase nor a decrease in the amount of the tumor by more than 25%.

Stage: The depth and extent of the cancer. The stages of bladder cancer are set forth in the TNM staging system. *See chapter 5, figures 5.1 and 5.2. See also* **TNM staging system**

Staging: The process of determining the stage (depth and extent) of the cancer.

Standard of care: A treatment that experts agree is appropriate, accepted, and widely used. Also called *standard treatment.*

Standard treatment. *See* **Standard of care**

Stoma. *See* **Ostomy**

Stoma catheter: A *stoma catheter* is inserted into a newly constructed continent catheterizable reservoir through an opening (stoma) in the abdominal wall. The purpose of the stoma catheter is to drain urine from the body while the continent catheterizable reservoir is healing. The stoma catheter is removed about 5 weeks after surgery.

Submucosa. See **Lamina propria**

Superficial bladder cancer: Non-muscle-invasive bladder cancer is sometimes called *superficial* bladder cancer. The term *superficial* can mask the seriousness of the disease, particularly if the cancer is high grade, which is an aggressive form of the disease.

Suprapubic catheter: Two catheters are inserted into a newly constructed continent catheterizable reservoir to drain urine while the body is healing: a *stoma* catheter and a *suprapubic* catheter, which is larger than the stoma catheter. The suprapubic catheter is used as a safety precaution in the event that the stoma catheter becomes clogged. After the stoma catheter is removed, the suprapubic catheter is left in place for about 2 more weeks. *See also* **Stoma catheter**

Surveillance: A disease is watched (monitored) during surveillance to detect any changes. During surveillance, tests and procedures are performed to evaluate the disease.

Systemic chemotherapy: The delivery of cancer-killing drugs into the bloodstream to treat cancer cells throughout the body. Systemic chemotherapy is given intravenously (into a vein) to treat patients with metastatic bladder cancer.

T

TIS (tumor in situ). *See* **Carcinoma in situ (CIS)**

Transitional cells. *See* **Urothelial cells**

Transitional cell carcinoma. *See* **Urothelial cell carcinoma**

Transitional epithelium. *See* **Bladder lining**

Transurethral resection. *See* **TUR** and **TURBT**

Transurethral resection of bladder tumor. *See* **TURBT** and **TUR**

TNM staging system: The system for staging bladder cancer. Uses the letters *T*, *N*, and *M* to indicate the location of the primary tumor (T), whether or not the tumor has metastasized (spread) to lymph nodes (N), and whether or not the tumor has metastasized to distant parts of the body (M). *See chapter 5, figure 5.2.*

Treatment plan: A plan for treatment that includes the names of drugs and dosages to be given and procedures to be performed, and the schedule and duration of treatment. Also referred to as *regimen* or *protocol.*

Trigone: The triangular-shaped area of the bladder where the ureters connect to the bladder. *See chapter 3, figures 3.6 and 3.7.*

Trimodality Therapy (TMT). *See* **Bladder Preservation Therapy**

Tumor: An abnormal mass of cells that results from uncontrolled cell division. A tumor with cancer cells present is called a *malignant* or *cancerous* tumor. A tumor with no cancer cells present is called a *benign* or *noncancerous* tumor. Also called *lesion.*

TUR. An acronym for TransUrethral Resection. *See* **TURBT**

TURBT. An acronym for TransUrethral Resection of Bladder Tumor. Also called **TUR** (TransUrethral Resection). During this procedure, a urologist passes an instrument, called a *resectoscope*, through the urethra to examine the lower urinary tract (bladder and urethra). The resectoscope is equipped with special tools for taking biopsies and removing (resecting) tumors. *See chapter 4, figure 4.2.*

U

Ultrasound: A type of imaging procedure that uses sound waves to create pictures of tissues and organs inside the body.

Unresectable: Cannot be removed surgically.

Upper urinary tract: The kidneys and ureters are in the upper urinary tract. *See chapter 3, figure 3.1(male) and 3.3 (female).*

Ureters: A pair of thin tubes — one on each side of the bladder — that carry urine from each of the kidneys to the bladder. *See chapter 3, figures 3.1 (male) and 3.3 (female).*

Urethral catheter. *See* **Foley catheter**

Urinalysis: A laboratory test to analyze the content of urine. Can detect bacteria and other abnormal substances in urine.

Urine culture: A laboratory test to check for bacteria, yeast, or other microorganisms in urine. This test can determine if blood in the urine is caused by a urinary tract infection, and, if so, the type of bacteria causing the infection.

Urine cytology: The microscopic examination of cells in a urine sample to determine if cancer is present in the bladder and/or other organs of the urinary tract. Also called *cytology.*

Urinary diversion. See **urinary tract reconstruction**

Urinary sphincter: Circular, donut-shaped muscles that control urine flow. There are two urinary sphincters, an involuntary (internal) sphincter and a voluntary (external) sphincter. When either sphincter contracts, it constricts the urethra and prevents urine from leaking. *See chapter 3, figures 3.2 (male) and 3.4 (female).*

Urinary system. *See* **Urinary tract**

Urinary tract: The function of the urinary tract is to filter out waste products from the blood and dispose of the waste in the form of urine, which ultimately is removed from the body. The organs of the urinary tract — the kidneys, ureters, bladder, and urethra — work together to produce, store, and excrete urine from the body. Also called *urinary system. See chapter 3, figures 3.1 (male) and 3.3 (female).*

Urinary tract infection (UTI): An infection in the urinary tract caused by bacteria that enters the urine and starts to grow. Common symptoms of a urinary tract infection are an urgent need to urinate, frequent urination, and pain or burning when urinating.

Urinary tract reconstruction: Reconstructive surgery performed during a radical cystectomy to provide a way for urine to leave the body after the bladder is removed. There are three types of urinary tract reconstructions: an ileal conduit, a neobladder, and a continent catheterizable reservoir. *See* **Ileal conduit**, **Neobladder**, and **Continent catheterizable reservoir**. Sometimes called *urinary diversion.*

Urologic oncology: A branch of medicine that specializes in the diagnosis and treatment of cancers of the male and female urinary tract (bladder, kidneys, ureters, urethra) and male reproductive system. Urologic oncology is a subspecialty of urology. Doctors who practice urologic oncology are called *urologic oncologists.*

Urology: A branch of medicine that specializes in the diagnosis and treatment of diseases of the male and female urinary tract and male reproductive organs. Medical specialists who practice urology are called *urologists.*

Urothelial cell carcinoma: Cancer that begins in the urothelial cells. Also called *transitional cell carcinoma.*

Urothelial cells: Cells that line the organs in the lower (bladder and urethra) and upper (kidneys and ureters) urinary tract. Also called *transitional cells.*

Urothelium. *See* **Bladder lining**

V

Vesical: A term that refers to the bladder.

Void: To empty the bladder by urinating.

INDEX

A

Adenocarcinoma, 52, 55
Adjuvant chemotherapy, 93
Anesthesia, general vs. spinal, 89
Anesthesiologist, 89, 164

B

BCG (bacillus Calmette-Guérin), 66, 67–68
Biopsy, 33, 34, 45
Bladder
    female, 23, 27
    function of, 21, 25
    location of, 25
    male, 22, 26
    structure of, 25, 28–29
Bladder cancer. *See also* Cell type;
    Diagnosis; Grade; Metastatic
    bladder cancer; Muscle-invasive
    bladder cancer; Non-muscle-
    invasive bladder cancer;
    Progression; Recurrence; Stage;
    Treatment options
    age and, 4, 162
    cell type of, 29, 52, 55
    gender and, 4, 162
    growth patterns of, 52–53
    health care professionals for,
     163–65
    prevalence of, 4
    risk factors for, 161–62
    symptoms of, 11, 35
    understanding "language" of, 9–10
Bladder lining, 28, 50, 51

Bladder preservation therapy
    candidates for, 123–27
    deciding on, 127–29
    follow-up care after, 131–32
    side effects of, 132
    three-pronged approach of, 77, 84,
     123, 129–31
Bladder-sparing therapy. *See* Bladder
    preservation therapy; Trimodality
    therapy (TMT)
Bladder wall, 28–29
Bladder wash, 38
Blood clots, avoiding, 110
Blue light cystoscopy, 34, 46, 65

C

Cancer survivor, definition of, 149.
    See also Survivorship care
Carboplatin, 139
Carcinoma in situ. *See* CIS
Catheterization, 103, 106
    self-, 102, 115
Catheters
    Foley, 112, 115
    stoma, 112, 115
    suprapubic, 112, 115
Cell type, 29, 52, 55
Chemoradiation, 84, 123, 130–31, 132
Chemotherapy. *See also*
    Chemoradiation
    adjuvant, 93
    intravesical, 66, 68
    neoadjuvant, 86–87
    systemic, 86–87, 93, 137–43

Cigarette smoking, 161

CIS (carcinoma in situ), 39, 50, 51, 53, 54, 55, 69–70, 125–26

Cisplatin, 126, 139

Clinical trials, 144–46

Continence, 30

Continent catheterizable reservoir, 103–6, 112, 115

CT (computed tomography) scan, 40–41

CT urogram (CTU), 41

Cure, definition of, 140

Cystoscope, 36, 37

Cystoscopy, 33, 36–37. *See also* Blue light cystoscopy

Cysview®, 46, 65

Cytology. *See* Urine cytology

Cystectomy. *See* Radical Cystectomy

Cytopathologist, 38, 164

D

da Vinci® Surgical System, 92

Diagnosis. *See also* Cell type; Grade; Second opinion; Stage
 of metastatic bladder cancer, 135–36
 of muscle-invasive bladder cancer, 73, 75–76
 of non-muscle-invasive bladder cancer, 61, 62–63, 68–71
 procedures and tests for, 33–34, 36–47
 understanding, 10, 49–56

Diet, 114, 162

Distant metastasis, 50, 51, 52, 136, 146

Doctors
 appointments with, 16–17
 choosing, 11–14
 communicating with, 10
 importance of relationship with, 10
 types of, 163–64

Drains, 110

E

Electrocauterization, 64

Enterostomal therapy (ET) nurse, 88, 96, 164. *See also* Ostomy nurse

Erectile dysfunction (ED), 117

Exercise, 114

F

Family history, 162

Fertility, 118

FISH, 39

Fluorescence cystoscopy. *See* Blue light cystoscopy

Foley catheter, 112, 115

Follow-up care plan, 153, 154–55

Fulguration, 64

G

GC regimen, 139

Gemcitabine, 139

Grade
 definition of, 49, 62
 low vs. high, 49–50, 53
 of muscle-invasive bladder cancer, 76
 of non-muscle-invasive bladder cancer, 62–63, 68, 69

H

Health care professionals, types of, 163–65

Hematuria, 11, 35
Hydronephrosis, 126

I
Ileal conduit, 96–99, 112–13, 119–22
Imaging tests, 33, 39–43
Immunotherapy
  for metastatic bladder cancer, 144
  for non-muscle-invasive bladder
    cancer, 66, 67–68
Incontinence, 99, 101, 102
Internet resources, 17
Intravesical chemotherapy, 66, 68
Intravesical drug therapy, 66–68
Intravesical immunotherapy, 66, 67–68

K
Kidneys, 21, 22, 23, 24–25

L
Lamina propria, 28, 50, 51
Lidocaine, 37
Locally advanced disease, 75
Lymphedema, 115
Lymph nodes, 31–32, 50, 51, 136

M
Medical oncologist, 13, 138–39, 164
Medical records
  keeping, 18–19
  obtaining copies of, 18, 57
Metastatic bladder cancer
  definition of, 135
  diagnosis of, 135–36
  palliative care for, 146
  staging system for, 54, 136–37
  treatment of, 137–46

Micrometastases, 86, 135–36
Micropapillary tumors, 53, 55
Mitomycin C, 66, 67, 68
MRI (magnetic resonance imaging),
  41–42
Mucosa, 28, 51
Muscle, 28, 29, 50, 51
Muscle-invasive bladder cancer
  definition of, 75
  grade of, 54, 76
  stages of, 54, 75–76
  treatment options for, 73, 77,
    79–93, 95–107, 109–32
Muscularis propria, 29, 51
MVAC regimen, 139

N
Neoadjuvant chemotherapy, 86–87
Neobladder, 99–103, 112, 115. *See also*
    Orthotopic neobladder
Non-muscle-invasive bladder cancer
  definition of, 61
  grades of, 54, 62–63, 68, 69
  monitoring of, 71–72
  progression of, 61, 63, 69, 70, 71
  recurrence of, 61, 63, 69, 70, 71
  stages of, 54, 62, 68–71
  treatment of, 63–68, 69, 70–71
Nurses
  enterostomal therapy (ET), 88, 96,
    164
  oncology, 165
  ostomy, 88, 96, 164

O
Oncologists
  medical, 13, 138–39, 164

radiation, 13, 164
urologic, 11–13, 138, 163–64
Oncology, definition of, 13
Oncology nurse, 165
Oncology social worker, 155, 165
Orthotopic neobladder, 99–103, 112, 115. *See also* Neobladder
Ostomy, definition of, 96
Ostomy bag, 96, 112–13, 120–22
Ostomy nurse, 88, 96, 164. *See also* Enterostomal therapy (ET) nurse

P
Pain, controlling, 110–11
Palliative care, 146
Papillary tumors, 52, 55
Partial cystectomy, 77, 83–84
Pathologist, 37, 164
Pathology report, 37, 56
postoperative, 93
Peristomal area, 120
Perivesical fat, 29, 51. *See also* Fat
PET-CT, 42–43
Primary care doctor, 163
Proactive patient, becoming, 5, 9–19, 155–57
Progression
definition of, 56, 63, 140, 151
of non-muscle-invasive bladder cancer, 61, 63, 69, 70, 71
risks of, 56, 152
Prostate, 22, 26, 30, 116, 117
Prostatic urethra, 22, 26, 29, 36

R
Radiation fields, 130
Radiation oncologist, 13, 164

Radiation therapy, 146. *See also* Chemoradiation
Radical cystectomy. *See also* Urinary tract reconstruction
alternatives to, 83–84
benefits of, 82
after bladder preservation therapy, 129
candidates for, 80–81
da Vinci® Surgical System and, 92
deciding on, 81–82
definition of, 30, 77, 79
fertility and, 118
follow-up care after, 115–16
home recovery after, 113–15
indications for, 80
postoperative hospital stay for, 109–11
postoperative pathology report after, 93
preparing for, 85–89
risks of, 83
sexual function and, 116–18
survival rates after, 82
undergoing, 89–93
Radiologist, 164
Radiosensitization, 130
Record of care, 153–54
Recurrence
definition of, 55, 63, 151
of non-muscle-invasive bladder cancer, 61, 63, 69, 70, 71
risks of, 55–56, 152
Remission
complete, 140
partial, 140
Resectoscope, 44, 64

Response
    complete, 131, 140
    definition of, 140
    partial, 140
    rate, 140
Restaging TURBT, 81
Risk factors, 161–62

S
Salvage radical cystectomy, 129
Sarcoma, 52, 55
Second cancer
    definition of, 152
    risks of, 152
Second opinion, 57, 81, 139
Self-catheterization, 102, 115
Sessile tumors, 53, 55
Sexual function, 116–18
Small cell carcinoma, 52, 55
Squamous cell carcinoma, 52, 55
Stable disease, definition of, 140
Stage
    definition of, 50, 62
    of metastatic bladder cancer,
        54–55, 136–37
    of muscle-invasive bladder cancer,
        54, 75–76
    of non-muscle-invasive bladder
        cancer, 54, 62, 68–71
    TNM staging system, 50–52,
        136–37
Stoma
    caring for, 119–20
    definition of, 96, 98, 105
    size of, 120
Submucosa, 28, 51
Support groups, 156

Supportive care, 146
Survivorship care
    creating plan for, 152–55
    questions and concerns for, 1
        49–52
    taking proactive role in, 155–57
Systemic chemotherapy, 137–43

T
Ta tumors, 50, 51, 54, 68–69
TIS. *See* CIS
T1 tumors, 50, 51, 54, 70–71
T2 tumors, 50, 51, 54, 75, 76
T3 tumors, 50, 51, 54, 75, 76
T4a tumors, 51, 54, 75, 76
T4b tumors, 51, 54, 76, 136
TNM staging system, 50–52, 136–37
Transitional epithelium, 28, 51
Transitional cell carcinoma, 52. *See*
    Urothelial cell carcinoma
Treatment facilities, choosing, 14
Treatment options
    bladder preservation therapy, 77,
        84, 123–32
    blue light cystoscopy, 65
    chemoradiation, 84, 123, 130–31
    clinical trials, 144–46
    intravesical chemotherapy, 66, 68
    intravesical drug therapy, 66–68
    intravesical immunotherapy, 66,
        67–68. *See also* BCG
    for metastatic bladder cancer,
        137–46
    for muscle-invasive bladder cancer,
        73, 77, 79–93, 95–107, 109–32
    for non-muscle-invasive bladder
        cancer, 63–68, 69, 71

partial cystectomy, 77, 83–84

radiation therapy, 146

radical cystectomy, 79–83, 85–93, 109–22

standard, 145

systemic chemotherapy, 137–43

TURBT, 63–64, 124–25, 130

understanding, 15–16

Trimodality therapy (TMT). *See* Bladder preservation therapy; Bladder-sparing therapy

TUR. *See* TURBT

TURBT (Transurethral resection of bladder tumor)

bladder preservation therapy and, 124–25, 130

complete, 124–25

as diagnostic procedure, 34, 44

radical cystectomy and, 80–81

restaging, 81

as treatment for non-muscle-invasive bladder cancer, 63–64

U

Ultrasound, 43

Ureters, 21, 22, 23, 24, 25

Urethra, 21, 22, 23, 29

Urinary diversion. *See* Urinary tract reconstruction

Urinary retention, 102

Urinary sphincters, 30–31

Urinary system

cancer in another part of, 152

components of, 21–29

function of, 21

Urinary tract reconstruction. *See also* Continent catheterizable reservoir; Ileal conduit; Orthotopic neobladder

choosing surgeon for, 106

choosing type of, 86, 95–106

definition of, 86

talking with other patients about, 106–7

Urine cytology, 38–39

Urine tests, 33, 38–39

Urologic oncologist, 11–13, 138, 163–64

Urologist, 11–12, 138, 163

Urothelial cell carcinoma, 29, 52–53, 55, 126–27, 152

Urothelium, 28, 50, 51

CPSIA information can be obtained
at www.ICGtesting.com
Printed in the USA
LVHW07s1239060718
582674LV00040B/461/P